HEALTHY AND FIT

A BEGINNER'S GUIDE TO DIET AND EXERCISE

RENEE CHATHAM, C.P.T

This Book is intended as a reference, not as a health manual to cure any diseases.
The information provided is designed to help you make informed decisions about your health.
It is not intended to substitute for any treatment you may have been prescribed by your doctor.
If you suspect that you have a medical problem, we encourage you to seek medical help.
The publisher advises readers to take full responsibility for their safety and know their limits.

The exercise and dietary programs in this book are not intended as a substitute for any exercise routine or dietary regimen that may have been prescribed by your doctor. As with any change in exercise and dietary programs, you should consult with your doctor or physician for approval before beginning a new program.

Mention of specific companies, organizations, or authorities in this book does not imply endorsement by the author, nor does it mention specific companies, organizations, or authorities imply that they endorse this book or its author.

This Book is dedicated to my husband, Ben. Without your guidance and support, this would not have been possible.

TABLE OF CONTENTS

Introduction

"I believe the greatest gift you can give yourself and your family is a healthy you."

Think about something that took you a long time to learn, perhaps as a young kid, riding a bike without the training wheels. I can remember being terrified to ride my bike without my training wheels in fear of falling, and having my friends making fun of me. But when I finally did, the greatest feeling was that accomplishment of knowing I could do it, and all of my fears vanished.

Most people today want to learn how to be healthier, but are unsure of how and where to start, especially with the age of technology and so much information out there that may or may not be accurate. It can get confusing and frustrating. First, understand why you want to make a change. Do you have a family history of heart disease, diabetes, or cancer, and want to be proactive in hindering these conditions from happening to you? Are you considered obese and want to be around for your family and children? These are questions you need to ask yourself.

Heart Disease

What is heart disease? Heart disease generally refers to conditions that involve narrowed or blocked blood vessels that can lead to heart attack, chest pain (angina), or stroke.

According to the *American Heart Association,* over 82 million Americans have heart disease. It is the number one leading cause of death. Each year more than 813,000 die from heart disease, which can be prevented by leading a healthy, active lifestyle.

Obesity

Dr. Cynthia Moore, MD, PhD for the CDC states, "One contributing factor is the fact that the way we eat has changed over the last 50 years. Americans are eating more processed foods and eating out more frequently. The foods offered in restaurants, snack shops, and in vending machines are higher is sugar, calories, and fat than what we typically prepare in our own homes. We are surrounded by food. We are constantly bombarded by it. We are consuming larger portion sizes and more calories than ever before."

While there is no one solution to this obesity epidemic we are facing, there are small steps we can take to resolve it. What can each of us do as individuals to be healthier? We can plan and prepare to choose better options suited for our needs; we can eat more vegetables and fruits and fewer foods high in sugar.

Everyone, including adults of all ages and children, need to get the recommended amount of physical activity.

As a Fitness Professional, I enjoy educating my clients on how they can be healthier; and I always stay up to date with the newest information. In 2014, I wrote an article for a local magazine about outdoor fitness. There are so many forms of fitness that you wouldn't see as exercise, and enjoy it! Not everyone wants to come to a gym for exercise, so I am always looking for alternatives to the gym to accommodate those individuals. I am very passionate about health and fitness, and want to share my experiences to continue to help others.

The Takeaway

My intentions in writing this eBook were to educate and inform those who want to choose a healthy lifestyle, but aren't sure where to go from there. My experience and education has brought me to today and wanting to help as many individuals as I can. As you go through chapter by chapter, the information provided will give you a better understanding of what health and fitness is, and ways you can improve upon your life for the better. No two people are the same, but we all have a similar goal in mind; **to be happy and healthy!**

Chapter 1

Fitness at any Age

"You are never too old to set another goal or to dream a new dream." ~ C.S. Lewis

In my profession as a fitness trainer and instructor, I work with a variety of individuals of all ages ranging from age 6 to 85. Getting the recommended amount of physical activity for all these different groups is vital for overall health.

2008 Physical Activity Guidelines for Americans

These guidelines are needed because of the importance of physical activity to the health of Americans, whose current inactivity puts them at risk. Substantial health benefits are gained by doing physical activity according to the Health.Gov Guidelines presented below for the different age groups.

Children and Adolescents (6-17)

1. Children and adolescents should do 1 hour (60 minutes) or more of physical activity every day.

2. Most of the 1 hour or more a day should either be moderate or vigorous intensity aerobic activity.

3. As part of their daily physical activity, children and adolescents should do vigorous intensity activity on at least 3 days per week. They should also do muscle strengthening and bone strengthening activity on at least 3 days per week.

Adults (18-64)

1. Adults should do 2 hours and 30 minutes a week of moderate intensity, or 1 hour and 15 minutes (75 minutes) a week of vigorous intensity aerobic activity, or an equivalent combination of moderate to vigorous intensity activity. Aerobic activity should be performed in episodes of at least 10 minutes, preferably spread throughout the week.

2. Additional health benefits are provided by increasing to 5 hours (300 minutes) a week of moderate activity, or 2 hours and 30 minutes a week of vigorous intensity activity, or an equivalent of both.

3. Adults should also do muscle strengthening activities that involve all major muscle groups performed on 2 or more days per week. Muscles consisting of chest, back, shoulders, biceps, triceps, abdominal, and legs in general.

Older Adults (65+)

Older adults should follow the adult guidelines. If this is not possible due to limiting chronic conditions, older adults should be physically active as their abilities allow.

You should avoid inactivity. Older adults should do exercises to improve balance if they are at risk of falling.

The Health Benefits of Physical Activity

Scientific evidence suggests that physical activity helps lower the risk of heart disease, stroke, type 2 diabetes, high blood pressure, weight loss when combined with diet, improved cardiorespiratory fitness, reduces depression, and lowers the risk of early death.

Regular physical activity can improve your muscle strength and endurance. Exercise delivers oxygen and nutrients to your tissues and helps your cardiovascular system work more efficiently. And when you heart and lungs work more efficiently, you have more energy to go about your daily activities of living.

Key Guidelines for Safe Physical Activity

Understand the risks and be assured that physical activity is safe for almost everyone. Choose types of activities that are appropriate for your current fitness level and goals. Increase physical activity gradually over time, "start low and go slow". If you have chronic conditions or injuries you should always consult with your healthcare provider about any type and amount of activity appropriate for you.

Make Exercise Fun!

No matter what age, fitness should not be a chore. If you cringe at the notion of exercising, there are many activities that are fun and you wouldn't even know they count as exercise. I have provided a list below of a few activities you may want to consider if your current health status allows:

1. **Dancing**. Yes dancing! From ballroom dancing, line dancing, to even hip hop dancing. It all counts as exercise. A great calorie burner for sure!

2. **Hiking**. If you love the outdoors, this is top on my personal list. I could hike for hours. I love taking pictures of nature, so this one doesn't even seem like exercise to me. It can be a great family adventure.

3. **Jump Rope**. The jump rope is a great all around tool to help with balance and coordination, while working the muscles groups in your arms, legs, abdomen, and shoulders.

4. **Riding a Bicycle**. This is also a great exercise for the entire family. I reside in a state where families are active, especially outdoors.

5. **Tennis**. You could potentially burn up to 600 calories per hour playing tennis. This is a great cardiovascular exercise combined with strength training for the legs, arms, and upper body.

All of the above are intended as suggestions only. You are responsible for knowing your limitations. Always consult with your Physician before starting a new program.

Get Moving!

You may have heard the term, *"Use it or lose it"*, which by definition means that if you don't continue to practice or use your ability, you might lose that ability.

Sedentary lifestyles are harming Americans. Lack of physical activity can lead to an increased risk in certain cancers, type 2 diabetes, high blood pressure, heart disease, and even death.

The simplest, positive change you can make to improve your health is walking, and it's free! 30 minutes a day in 5 days is a realistic goal to start with. You can also divide the 30 minutes a day into increments, 10 minutes at a time.

Everyone has to start somewhere. Even if you have been inactive for many years, today is the day where you begin your journey to make healthy changes in your life. Something is always better than nothing!

Chapter 2

Getting Started

"The expert at anything was once a beginner." ~ Helen Hayes

So, you've decided it's time to start exercising and eating healthy. Congratulations! This is a great step to a new you. Now you may be wondering, "What do I do now or, how do I start?"

Setting Goals

This should be your first step. Setting goals are a plan of action taken to guide you through this journey. It gives you the ability to be in control of your life. You can visualize your ideal end goal and turn it into reality. Goal setting helps you achieve what you set out to do, one step at a time.

When you set a goal or goals, it becomes your starting point to success. You now have the motivation to achieve what is important to you.

SMART Goals

SMART is an acronym for the 5 steps of *Specific, Measurable, Attainable, Realistic,* and *Timely.* A SMART goal provides an individual with more direction and a better ability to achieve the goal by the targeted complete date.

1. **Specific**- This is your detailed description of what it is to be accomplished. Take into consideration a few questions when setting theses specific goals:

-What is my objective (goal)?

-What is my target date to complete my goal?

-What is my reason or purpose for accomplishing my goal?

For example, let's say you want to lose weight. Saying I want to lose weight is vague, so instead put a number on the weight you would like to lose and the time frame in which this is to be accomplished, along with why you want to accomplish this.

"I want to lose 15 pounds in 10 weeks so that my bridesmaid dress fits me perfectly."

2. **Measurable**- Capable of being measured. A measurable goal will usually answer questions of how much, how many, and how will I know it is accomplished.

If the specific goal is to lose 15 pounds and the time frame is 10 weeks, to measure your progress you would use a weight scale to determine if you are reaching your goal.

3. **Attainable**- When you identify goals that are important to you, this is when you begin to find ways to make those goals come true. Attainable goals are those of the right mix that are challenging, but not extreme. An attainable goal will usually be one that is realistic, able to

be reached in the period of time you are working towards.

4. **Realistic**- What does it mean to be realistic? The following will help you identify if you can achieve your goal:

-Am I being sensible? Is this goal able to be achieved in my time frame?

-Am I willing to put the effort in? Is this something I can commit to?

-Do I believe I can do this (even if it is hard)?

To be realistic, a goal must represent an objective toward which you are both willing and able to work at. A goal is probably realistic if you truly believe it can be accomplished.

5. **Timely**- Every goal needs to have a specific date in which you want to complete it. The time should not be too distant into the future. For example, set goals that can be achieved tomorrow and in 3 months.

Now that you have an idea of your starting point with setting your goal(s), I will provide a template on the following page.

"Setting a goal is not the main plan. It is deciding how you will go about achieving it and staying with it."

Table 2.1 below is a general outline to help you write out your goal(s) and reference back to as you continue with your journey to a healthier you.

Table 2.1		

SMART GOALS OUTLINE

SPECIFIC Your detailed description of the goal.	What do you want to accomplish?	Notes:
MEASURABLE How you will track your progress.	How will you know when the goal is accomplished?	Notes:
ATTAINABLE Are you committed to completing the goal?	How can the goal accomplished?	Notes:
REALISTIC Is this a goal you are able to finish?	Is the goal reasonable?	Notes:
TIMELY Set a date for the completion. This keeps you motivated.	What timeframe do I want to complete my goal?	Notes:

The Benefits of Your Goal

There are many benefits to goal setting. The following is a list of just some of those benefits:

1. Goals direct attention to what is important to you.

2. It gives you direction, a path to follow, keeping you on track.

3. Empowerment. You are in control.

4. Self-Confidence. You are set out to do something good for yourself to feel better!

5. Increased Focus. With this goal in mind, you now have a reason to accomplish it.

6. Increased Motivation. When you are set out to do something, nothing will stop you from getting there. The greatest feeling is that of accomplishment.

7. You learn a lot about yourself. Whether you are setting a short term or long term goal, you will find out things about yourself you never knew, things you didn't know you were capable of. This is a growing process.

The Mind is a Powerful Thing

So, we've established our aspiring goals, now do we have our mind set to achieve them? In this next section, I want to discuss the stages of change, and the psychological aspects before beginning a new program.

The Stages of Change

Take a moment to reflect back upon a diet or health behavior you attempted to change in the past, but did not stick with for a long period of time. Identify your primary reason or reasons you believe may have attributed to this lack of success. Was it lack of motivation? Too challenging or complicated? Did you have too many distractions that caused you to lose focus? Was your lack of knowledge a contributing factor? Maybe you weren't ready at the time. Now let's discuss the stages of change.

Stage 1: PRECONTEMPLATION

Individuals in the first stage have no intentions to make any changes in the immediate future. Why? They may not be fully aware of all the potential benefits, may have attempted in the past and became frustrated and gave up, or lack of energy to not want to make the effort.

"Several times in my career I have witnessed family members attempting to "change" one another by suggesting an exercise program. If one family member isn't quite ready for the "change", there isn't anything that can be done to say otherwise. If they don't want to do it, they won't do it, or it creates resentment in the future."

Stage 2: CONTEMPLATION

Those in this stage of contemplation are thinking about taking action, but aren't quite ready or don't know how to get started. Contemplators often think they might make changes with the next six months, and they are open to information and feedback. However, they are on the fence, so to speak. Maybe someone suggested a fitness class to them, and while it sounds like it could be a good idea, they aren't 100% sure about doing it.

Stage 3: PREPARATION

This is the stage in which an individual is getting ready to take action. They are more decisive and committed; they are developing a plan and may have already taken small steps to start. At this point, the pros of making a change clearly outweigh the cons. At this stage you should be encouraged to pick a specific day on which you will officially begin your planned stage.

"Clients come to me when they are in this stage of preparation. They are determined to make a change for the better. They might be at a point where they can no longer live the way they are living, and have decided to finally set that goal to achieve."

Stage 4: ACTION

This is the stage where an individual has begun doing something, but have not been consistent for over 6 months. It is vital in this action stage to not lose sight of the goal. Making your choices a part of your everyday lifestyle and staying accountable for your actions.

Stage 5: MAINTENANCE

Individuals in this stage have maintained for over 6 months. They have successfully avoided or have overcome any obstacles that could have caused them to regress back to old behaviors or habits. Their new behaviors have now become an important part of their lifestyle and identity.

Yet, several things could cause a relapse: stress, boredom, lack of environmental or emotional support, or a frustrating plateau. Major life events- like a job change, loss of a family member, a romantic breakup, relocation, birth of a child can also cause trigger a relapse.

"Typically when I see people in the maintenance stage, they are pretty well set with continuing to succeed. There can be setbacks yes, but if you set your mind to do something, nothing will stop you in the long term. Everyone has a bad day; just don't let it affect the future."

Now that we have discussed the stages of change, take a moment to see where you are in these stages. Are you in contemplation or preparation? Now think about where you would like to be, action or maintenance, and now you can take the necessary steps to get there.

Chapter 3

Exercise at Home vs a Gym

"To enjoy the glow of good health, you must exercise." ~Gene Tunney

If you are new to exercise and have some health concerns, it is recommended that you consult with your doctor prior to beginning any fitness program.

Decisions, Decisions

Now that you have your goal set in mind, do you exercise at home or at a gym? Both have their pros and cons. There could be many things that could play a factor when deciding if a going to a gym or exercising at home is right for you.

Let's first discuss the pros of a home work out:

1. *It is convenient.* You don't have leave the comfort of your home, you could exercise in your pajamas if you want to!

2. *Small children at home.* You don't have to worry about childcare, as most gyms only have a set time when they have daycare.

3. *Quick workout.* You never have to wait for equipment like you would at a busy gym.

4. *Free.* You can do all body weight exercises and it's free!

5. *Time*. You can exercise at any time you wish.

6. *Saves drive time and money*. You have to drive 10 to 20 minutes to get to a gym and saves gas and miles on your vehicle.

Now you have a few pros to consider when deciding if exercise at home is right for you.

Now let's discuss the cons of exercise at home:

1. *Lack of motivation*. I have seen this time and time again and I have even fell victim to it! You are able to exercise in the comfort of your own home, but don't feel like it. When you have somewhere to go to exercise, or have a work out buddy, you are more likely to have the motivation to workout.

2. *Not having all the equipment of gym*. It makes it a little hard to mix up your workout when you don't have equipment at home, or have the line of equipment a gym has.

3. *Equipment is costly*. If you purchase a home gym, which are typically in the thousands in cost, not everyone can afford to pay up front.

4. *Too many distractions*. Most families today have children and pets, and even parents living with them. It can make it difficult to get an effective workout in when kids are calling for you, or the dog(s) need to go outside!

5. *Maintenance*. If you do purchase equipment, you are responsible for the cost of repair.

6. *Space*. Not everyone has the luxury of a full basement or a large home capable of a storing all the equipment you may need.

Certified Personal Trainer Laurette Schroeck provided an insight on working out at home. Here's what she had to say:

"The biggest pro to working out at home is convenience. Sometimes with work, children or other commitments it's hard to physically get to a gym sometimes which is why I really enjoy working out at home. I can do it whenever I want, whether it's first thing in the morning or at the end of the night. When I started as a beginner, I really enjoyed working out at home because I felt comfortable, whereas at a gym I would feel intimidated by others around me. If I needed to stop and take a break I could, if I needed to stop early because I felt I couldn't push myself anymore I could and I didn't feel like I had eyes on me and I didn't feel judged, so it was a more comfortable situation. However, once advancing to an intermediate level of fitness compared to a beginner, I started to lose motivation. I realized I started to need to be around more people to motivate me and push me. Physically going to the gym made me feel more accountable and it also gave me access to a bigger variety of tools to help me along the way, whereas at home I was more limited."

Advantages of exercise at a gym:

1. *Variety of equipment.* What I always look for in a gym is a really good variety of equipment. The more options the better, especially if get bored easy.

2. *Group classes.* If you enjoy interacting with others, group classes are great! Group classes provide a positive atmosphere and you tend to be very motivated than if you were to exercise on your own.

3. *Guidance.* Most gyms provide personal trainers to assist in helping you with exercise and how to use the equipment.

4. *Atmosphere.* You tend work harder when people are around you at the gym. Others may motivate you to do more.

5. *Time for yourself.* You have the much needed time away from distractions, a ringing phone, screaming kids, etc.

Disadvantages of exercise at a gym:

1. *Cost.* Typically gym memberships can range from $20-$100 or more depending on type, location, amenities, etc.

2. *Drive time.* Unless your gym is 5 minutes away, you could spend 10-20 minutes to get to the gym.

3. *Germs!* There have been several times in the years I have been going to the gym that I caught someone's cold. Not everyone has the best hygiene habits.

4. *Being watched*. If you aren't one for being looked at while working out, you may be intimidated by people at a gym.

5. *Waiting for machines*. Depending on the time of day you work out, there are typical "busy" times in which there is an influx of people, before work, after kids go to school, after work, etc.

A gym can be an intimidating place if you are a beginner. But after a few work outs, you should begin to feel like one of the regulars.

If you are considering the gym route, here are a few things to keep in mind when finding the right gym for you:

1. *Location*. If the gym isn't located close to your home or work, you are less likely to go.

2. *Amenities*. If you are a parent of a small child, a daycare at gym is a must for you. If you love to swim, you may want a gym that has an indoor pool. The gym that accommodates to your needs is what you should consider.

3. *Hours*. Is the gym 24 hours? Not everyone has the same schedule and could have odd hours for working. A gym that has hours within you are able to go is best.

4. *Group Classes*. Not everyone wants to lift weights or just do cardio and may need motivation or instruction and prefer group classes. Does the gym have classes you like or would try?

5. *Comfort*. When you walk into a gym for the first time, do you feel overwhelmed by the amount of equipment and/or people? Sometimes choosing a smaller gym may be a great place to start, so there is no intimidation or anxiety.

6. Lastly, *Cost*. I say this last when deciding on a gym because when you are set on beginning your new journey, money should only factor a small amount in your decision. Most gyms are very competitive, especially in price. When you have a gym with much more amenities to offer, the cost reflects it.

Let's do this!

The time to start is now! Hopefully you have a little more information you may not have had before you started reading this. As we move in to the next chapter, I will discuss what a workout consists of and choosing the options that work well for you. Not everyone has the exact same capabilities, so it is important to understand where you are, where you want to be, and how you plan to get there.

Chapter 4

Anatomy of a Workout

"When you put the time and effort in preparing for the task at hand, you have a greater chance of making it happen."

Prepare for your workout

Before you even begin your new exercise program, it is important to be prepared so you have continued success. If you have everything you need and know what you will be doing, you are more likely to complete the goal. Here are a few steps to begin:

1. **Schedule your workout**. Time is the #1 excuse used by people on why they do not exercise. Make the time in your busy day and put in on your calendar until you have a routine and it becomes second nature.

2. **Have workout gear ready**. A big time saver! Always have your clothes out the night before. Then you aren't wasting time wondering what you will wear. If you are going to exercise after work and are unable to go back home, pack a gym bag.

3. **Plan what you will do**. You should already have an idea of what form of exercise you will do on a given day. If you are working out at home, write down the exercises in the order you wish to perform them in. You can do the same

if you are going to the gym. Is cardio on your list? Write down the form of cardio you plan on doing. For example; Treadmill for 30 minutes, then elliptical for 15 minutes on Monday.

Know what muscles you are working

Before we discuss the actual workouts, I want to provide a short anatomy lesson you may or may not already be familiar with. While there are many muscles in the human body, I will only be discussing a few:

1. *Deltoid*- this is the shoulder. You have 3 parts to your deltoid, the anterior (front shoulder), medial, (side), and posterior (back).

> *Exercises*: Shoulder press, lateral raises, front raises, reverse fly, Arnold press, and upright row.

2. *Latissimus Dorsi or "Lats"*- The widest portion of your back, when you lift weights, it creates that nice "V" shape.

> *Exercises*: Pull downs, pull ups, straight arm pull down,   seated row.

3. *Pectoralis Major or "Pecs"*- This is your main chest muscle.

> *Exercises*: Bench press, push-ups, cable fly

4. **Biceps**- the muscle that lies on the upper arm between your shoulder and elbow. You have 2 parts to the bicep, short head and long head ("bi" meaning 2).

Exercises: Bicep Curl, Concentration Curl, hammer curl, preacher curl.

5. **Triceps**- the back of the upper arm, some older folks, in fun, call these "bat wings". The triceps have 3 parts, the short head, long head, and medial head ("tri" meaning 3).

Exercises: Triceps dumbbell kickback, dips, skull crushers, close grip barbell press, push down, triceps overhead press.

6. *Rectus Abdominis or "Abs"*- this is your center, or "core". This is where you may have heard the term six pack, when the abdominal muscles are visible.

Exercises: Crunches, leg raises, plank.

7. *Quadriceps or "Quads"*- You have 4 muscles in your upper front thigh (quad meaning 4, isn't that neat!)

Exercises: leg extension, lunges, jump squats, leg press

8. *Hamstrings*- This would refer to the back of the upper thigh. There are also 4 different muscles in the hamstring complex.

Exercises: leg curl, stiff leg deadlift, box jump, knee tuck jump

9. *Glutes or "buttocks"*- You have 3 specific muscles that make up your backside; gluteus maximus, gluteus medius, and gluteus minimus.

Exercises: Floor bridge, squats, step-ups, glute kickbacks.

10. **Calves**- The main muscles that create that "heart" shape in the back of your lower leg are the gastrocnemius and soleus.

> *Exercises*: Standing or seated calf raises, sprints, cycling, jumping rope

The Warm up:

The first component of a workout should be to prepare the muscles for exercise; this is where the warm up comes in. A proper warm up can increase blood flow to the working muscles which results in decreased muscle stiffness, less risk of injury, and improved performance.

The purpose of a warm up includes: increasing range of motion of joints, gradually increase body temperature and heart rate, plus it is a good form of mental preparation. Your mind can ease into the workout.

Aerobic exercise

Aerobic exercise, also known as cardio, is one way to incorporate a warm up. A brisk walk, either outside or on a treadmill for 5-7 minutes is a great way to prepare the body for exercise. For the treadmill setting for beginners, I typically recommend setting the speed to 3.0 to start, and slowly work your way up.

Dynamic Stretching

Dynamic stretching is a type of stretching where you are providing movement of the muscle, but not holding at the end motion. Examples of dynamic stretching include: high knees, arm circles, butt kicks, skipping, shoulder rolls, etc.

Dynamic stretches can also mimic the exercises you intend to perform. Examples may be: body squats, jump squats, side bends, walking lunges, etc.

It is recommended to perform about 5 minutes of dynamic stretching with 10-15 repetitions each movement.

I instruct group fitness classes for the older population, and I wanted to share a typical warm up I use for my class:

Neck Rolls- 10 repetitions

Shoulder Rolls forward/ back- 10 repetitions each

Arm circles forward/back- 10 repetitions each

Side bends- 10 repetitions each side

Torso twist- 10 repetitions each way

Lateral lunge side to side- 10 repetitions

High knees- 15 each leg

Step side to side- 10 repetitions

Walk in place- 20 seconds

For a beginner, these are the two forms of warm ups I recommend to any individuals who are just starting out.

Different types of training

Circuit: A circuit training workout is one that works each section of the body individually. You would move from exercise to exercise with little rest in between. You may choose a circuit to target upper body one day and lower body the next, or train the entire body.

The typical sets you would perform would be low to moderate in number (1-3), with moderate to high repetitions (8-20), and short rest time (15-60 seconds)

Benefits of Circuit Training

A few benefits of the circuit training workout it is both a cardiovascular and muscular workout rolled into one. It gets the heart rate up, burns fat, and tones the body. It can also be great for individuals who get bored easy with working out. You are always moving and doing different exercises. For beginner's, this is a great place to start.

The Circuit Training Workout

Now that you have a concept of circuit training is, now you may be wondering, "What do I do now?" I am here to help:

1. Always start with your *warm-up*. You can do a cardio warm up and/or a dynamic warm up.

2. Next, a *total body exercise*, examples are: Sumo squat to upright row with a kettlebell, step up to front or lateral raise, ball squat, bicep curl to overhead press.

3. If you are new to exercise and unfamiliar with an order in which to do your exercises, an order I have been taught and use for myself is: chest, back, shoulders, biceps, triceps, and legs. While there are many different ways to train, I have found this to be a great way to achieve muscle tone in a short amount of time.

Example*: Chest press, pull-up, reverse fly, bicep curl, triceps press down, leg press.*

Remember- You are doing 1 set with anywhere from 8-10 repetitions. You can repeat the circuit one or two more times if you would like.

Split Routine: This type of training involves breaking up the body parts on separate days. For example, Monday you could do chest, back, and shoulders, Tuesday is your Leg workout, and Thursday you work your biceps and triceps.

For those new to this type of training, the typical adequate starting point is 2-3 sets with 10-12 repetitions.

You would complete the sets for the same exercise before moving on to the next exercise.

Benefits of Split Training

Several benefits that stand out with split routine training is you are able to focus on a specific body part, overload that body part, and have increased muscle strength and mass in a short amount of time. You are less likely to fatigue versus circuit training. If your goal is to get muscular, this is a great training style to achieve that. You are also able to train several days in a row when you split upper and lower body, reaching that goal sooner.

The Cool Down

Now that you understand your warm up and your options for exercise, we will discuss the final component to your workout, the cool down. The purpose of a cool down is to bring the heartrate back down to normal and to get the blood circulating freely back to the heart. A slow pace walk or slow pace on the recumbent bicycle for 5-10 minutes are a couple examples.

Stretches

Take the time to stretch at the end of your workout. This allows you to relax and stretch out all the major muscles you've just used. Stretching may help reduce muscle fatigue and soreness. You also have an increase in flexibility when you have properly stretched post workout.

Below I will provide examples of stretches I use every day with clients:

1. **Shoulder stretch**- Cross one arm in front of your body (horizontal) touching your opposite shoulder, and pressing with the other arm into the elbow. The best way to describe this stretch is, "you're giving yourself a hug".

2. **Triceps stretch-** Starting with your right arm, extend arm straight up, then bending at the elbow placing your hand behind your head, reach with the left hand to your right elbow, gently press back on your elbow.

Biceps stretch- Place arms straight out to your sides, rotate your arms back, pointing your thumbs back, hold the stretch, return back to the starting position, and repeat.

Chest stretch- Clasp hands back behind you, gently pressing down and back bringing your shoulders back and chest out. This also stretches the front of the shoulder.

Back stretch- For those with back discomfort, you can use a chair to stretch. Depending on your height, stand about 3-4 feet away from a chair, reaching towards the chair keeping the arms straight, hinging forward from the hip. If you do not feel a stretch, step back from the chair a little further.

Quadricep stretch (front thigh) - Two options for this stretch seated or standing. For seated, sit to one side of your chair, extend the leg this is at the other most side, until you feel a stretch in your front thigh. Repeat on other side. For standing, bring leg up behind you, grab at your ankle and hold.

Hamstring stretch (back of the thigh) - Standing upright, reach down towards your feet. The key is to keep legs straight, but if you have tightness in the hamstring, you tend to bend slightly at the knee. If you cannot reach to your toes, that is okay.

Calf stretch- Place hands on a wall, extending right leg back, keeping the right leg straight and heel on the floor, bend left knee in. Repeat on other side.

Adductor stretch (side lunge)- With a wide stance, bend one leg at a 90 degree angle, keeping the opposite leg straight, placing your hand(s) on the bent knee. Repeat on other side. This will stretch out your inner thigh.

How long to hold each stretch

To achieve the greatest benefits for flexibility you should hold each stretch for a maximum of 30 seconds. Typically 20-30 seconds is best. This type of stretching is what is referred to as "static stretching." Static stretching exercises are used for a cool down to help improve mobility and range of motion.

While there are other forms of stretching, I wanted to begin with basics, great for beginners. Starting something new can be an overwhelming process; rather than create a sense of confusion or frustration, let's create a program that is easy to remember and follow.

Avoid Overtraining

As a fitness professional, I have seen individuals, especially those who have a new found love of exercise, taking it to extremes. I am guilty of this as well. You start to exercise, see results, and next thing you know you aren't giving your body a break. You are exercising every day, even twice a day. You become obsessed. This is not good for your overall health. I want to discuss the signs and symptoms of overtraining and how to avoid putting your health in harm's way.

The Signs and Symptoms

1. *Constant muscle soreness*: You always feel sore, even if you didn't work that body part for several days.

2. *Irritability*: You get agitated very easy, every little thing sets you off.

3. *Increased incidence of injuries*: You are constantly pushing your body to the limits, resulting in a higher likelihood of injury.

4. *You are always exhausted*: Exercise should help you feel energized. After your workout you may be tired, since you put forth the effort, but that feeling should diminish. If you are sluggish throughout your entire day, your body may be telling you something.

5. *Always getting sick*: You may feel like you have a persistent cold that just won't go away. Your immune system is giving 100% to fight off that cold or flu.

6. *Insomnia*: You may have difficulty falling asleep or have restless sleep. Your body is in recovery mode when you are at rest. A body that is overtraining sometimes is unable to slow down and completely relax.

While these are just a few signs and symptoms of overtraining, it is important to give your body rest. Take a break from exercise for a short time to allow healing. Your body will thank you!

In Conclusion

Finding a fitness program that suits your needs is the key. What works for a *20 year old* may not work for *a 50 year old* that may have had back surgery or knee surgery. Know your limitations and how to work around them.

Starting a new exercise program is a big first step. It can be intimating when you are not sure if you are doing everything correctly. In this chapter, I have provided a basic outline of a simple workout. In the next chapter, I will discuss the personal training aspect, and if working with a trainer is right for you.

Chapter 5

Should I hire a Personal Trainer?

What is a Personal Trainer?

A personal trainer is a fitness professional possessing the knowledge, skills and abilities to provide safe and effective exercise and fitness program design, instruction and assistance for the purpose to help others reach their personal health and fitness goals. They provide motivation and education to help you achieve success.

6 Reasons you should hire a personal trainer

More and more people in need of guidance are looking to a personal trainer for assistance. In my experience as a certified personal trainer, everyone has a different reason for hiring a fitness professional for guidance. I will provide my opinion on how you know it is time to hire a professional.

1. ***You want to lose weight, but don't know how***. If your goal is to trim down your waistline, a personal trainer can help. They have the knowledge and training to kick your metabolism into high gear with exercises you probably didn't know existed. Some personal trainers also have a nutritional background to help you reach your goals.

2. ***You need to be motivated***. If you lack the motivation to exercise on your own, a trainer is there to inspire and motivate you. As you begin to see results, your motivation will increase and the likelihood that you'll exercise on your own is greater.

3. ***You don't know where to start***. Typically, personal trainers also start with a consultation before they begin an exercise program with you. They will gather all the information that is critical in designing a program that fits your wants and needs. With their expertise, they should be able to guide you in the right direction for success.

4. ***You have a specific condition, illness, or injury***. Once you receive the okay from your doctor that you are able to exercise, working with an experienced trainer who has the ability to design a fitness program to help you prevent further injury or problems is crucial.

5. **You want to learn how to exercise correctly**. Hiring a personal trainer for at least a few sessions is a great benefit to learning the right way to exercise. A thorough personal trainer will explain what muscle is being worked, the name of the exercise, and correct form to reduce any risk of injury.

6. **You want to workout at home.** There are many personal trainers who will come to you for the workout. If you are like every other busy person out there, this is a huge plus. You don't need a gym membership and trainers who work for themselves can be less of cost since they aren't paying a portion of their earnings to a gym.

Certified Personal Trainer

A trainer that has successfully completed an accreditation program from a nationally recognized institution verifies the validity and competency that they have met the criteria to work as fitness *professional.* The NCCA is the National Commission for Certifying Agencies. The NCCA accredits programs that meet its standards. A few certification programs that are NCCA accredited are:

ACSM - *American College of Sports Medicine* Prerequisites to take the exam is age 18 or older, high school diploma or equivalent, and CPR with AED certification. The typical time frame one takes to study before taking the test is around 4 months. The ACSM certification examination is administered by computer at a testing facility not allowing for open book. Recertification is every 3 years, and requires continuing education credits to stay current.

NASM – *National Academy of Sports Medicine* Prerequisites to take the exam is age 18 or older, high school diploma or equivalent, and CPR with AED certification. NASM provides several study options for their aspiring personal trainers. The time frame for completion of this program is anywhere from 2 months to 6 months. The NASM certified personal trainer exam is also administered by computer at a testing facility. Recertification is every 2 years, and requires continuing education credits to remain certified.

ACE – *American Council on Exercise* Prerequisites to take the exam is age 18 or older and CPR with AED certification. The time frame can vary, but ACE allows up to 1 year completing their exam. The ACE exam is also administered by a testing facility. ACE requires recertification every 2 years along with continuing education credits to remain certified.

NSCA – *The National Strength and Conditioning Association* Prerequisites to take the exam is age 18 or older, high school diploma or equivalent, and CPR with AED certification. NSCA allows aspiring personal trainers to complete their certification within 6 months. Exams are administered by computer at testing centers across the United States. NSCA requires recertification every 2 years and continuing education credits to remain certified.

Is it important to hire a Certified Personal Trainer?

The short answer would be yes. Would you go to a regular physician if you needed heart surgery? No. This is why there are specialists out there for this reason. You can hire someone who "trains" people and isn't certified to be a personal trainer, but do they have complete knowledge of what is required to provide safe and effective training? You can be the judge of that.

A qualified personal trainer has knowledge of basic exercise science, human movement science, specific fitness training (cardiovascular, strength, resistance, balance, core, flexibility, etc.) They provide you with a comprehensive fitness assessment to establish goals, your current level of fitness, body composition, etc. Hire a qualified trainer to get results.

Where do I find a Qualified Personal Trainer?

First ask family or friends if they have a recommendation for a personal trainer they may have used or a friend has used. You can ask your doctor as well; many doctors and physicians network with local trainers they might know and trust.

Next, you can research trainers in your area online. You can type "personal trainers" in the area you live. There are many sites that may show up or trainers that match your keywords.

Specific sites that provide several listings free for trainers are:

IDEA Health and Fitness Association: This is the largest network to find a certified personal trainer. You can search by the city in which you reside, whether you want a male or female trainer, the cost you are looking for, and even specific specialties, such as bodybuilding.

Personaltrainer.com: This site isn't as widely known as IDEA, but another great resource. Trainers create a listing for their area and provide a lot of information so that you can choose the right person for you.

iPersonaltrainer.net: Another great resource to finding a certified personal trainer within your area. This is similar to the site mentioned above, as the trainer provides a detailed description on his or hers services.

Thumbtack: This site is where personal trainers "bid" for your business. You provide a listing of the services you are in search of, example, need a Female personal trainer, Goals: weight loss and nutrition, your age, preferred location to train, times and days to train, etc.

The Cost of a Personal Trainer

Cost will always vary. It depends on location, the trainer's experience, their specialties, if they train at a gym versus in home training. They may base their fees on a session to session rate, monthly rate, or package rate. The higher of a commitment you are willing to make (2 months or more of training or 3 days a week versus 1 day a week) the lesser cost breakdown per session, respectively.

How to Decide Who is Right for You

Before you choose a trainer, here are few things to consider:

1. **Experience** - If you are looking to lose weight, you may choose a trainer who has a specialty in weight loss. Their site may have testimonials or success stories of people who have lost weight.

2. **Availability** – Are they able to perform training sessions when it is convenient for you? Trainers don't have a typical 9-5 job schedule. They are flexible with your schedule and should accommodate to you.

3. **Cost** – Are the fees within your budget and what you are willing to pay? Just because a trainer has a very low

rate doesn't mean much. They could be new to training or have little to no overhead so they can pass on the savings to you. Also, if a trainer's rate is high, doesn't mean they are better than the lower cost trainer.

4. **Personality** – You might be working with this person for an extended period of time. It is very important they have a personality that matches your needs. You need to be able to build a trusting relationship with the trainer, so if your personalities don't mesh or there is a lack of communication it will never work.

5. **Professionalism** – While it is important for a trainer to develop a relationship with their client, there also needs to be a level of professionalism. Rude or inappropriate comments can make you feel uncomfortable and can discourage you, and then you lose confidence in yourself.

6. **Appearance** – You want a trainer who presents themselves in such a way that you have all the confidence in the world that they will get you to your goal. A trainer who has a sloppy appearance could say many things; they may not care too much about their look, or maybe they don't take much time putting themselves together every day. While appearances aren't everything, wouldn't you have more trust in a trainer who takes care of themselves to help you become successful?

Interview the Trainer

The first meeting with the potential trainer you want to hire should determine if they are right for you. While this is the time they will be asking you many questions, do not be afraid to ask them questions as well. You are the one who will be paying for their services, so ask all the questions you need to get the all the answers to help you determine if he or she is right for you:

1. *How long have you been a trainer?* While this isn't 100% what you should base your decision on, it is good to know how much experience the trainer has had. Maybe you have had a knee replacement; a trainer who has been training for some time or has specialties in injuries and prevention, would be a good fit for you.

2. *What Certifications do you have?* Always hire a trainer who has had specific training to become a fitness professional. As I had mentioned prior, a certification is a credential given by an agency or institution with its own educational and testing procedures. Quality agencies (NCCA) require a thorough process of certifying trainers. There are many agencies on the internet that "sell" personal training courses, but the standards are not as high as those through courses that are approved through the *National Commission for Certifying Agencies* (NCCA) which states the standards were developed to ensure the health, welfare, and safety of the public. You will want to also ask that they have their Cardiopulmonary resuscitation (CPR) through an accredited training course; American Heart Association or Red Cross, as examples.

3. *How often should I train?* Based on the goals you outline to the trainer, they should be able give you recommendations based on those goals, your fitness level, and commitment. If you are brand new to exercise, they may recommend starting out with two days a week. You may be given "homework" to do outside of the training sessions with the fitness professional.

4. *What is the cost?* You will need to determine if the training rates are within your budget. Remember, this is a commitment to your health. Choosing a trainer based just on rates isn't always going to get you the results that you want and need. Experienced trainers will always have a slightly higher rate.

5. *Do you offer a session for free?* Not all trainers offer a session for free. It is not a bad thing if they don't. I personally didn't start out giving sessions for free, but I did give deep discounts. As I have grown as a trainer, I now provide a first free session just to give my potential client an idea of what is like to train with me. They can then base their decision on if my training style suits their needs.

Making the Decision

If you find it difficult to exercise on your own or have trouble staying motivated, a personal trainer is there to assist you in all of these things. You may have short term goals that you need to accomplish, and without the help of a fitness professional, you may not achieve those goals. Decide if hiring a trainer is right for you.

Chapter 6

Design Your Own Workout

You can do it!

Now you have decided you want to design a workout on your own. With all of the resources out there, you don't feel the need to hire a trainer to help you reach your goals. You feel pretty confident you can do it on your own. Maybe you have a little knowledge on exercise, or you've played sports in high school and understand how to exercise. It is always a good to use resources to try new things and see if they work for you.

In this chapter, We will define the myths versus truths about diet and exercise, provide examples of workouts for home and the gym, a breakdown of exercises and how to do them using proper form, and all the steps to help you become successful in your journey to health and fitness.

Myths Vs Truths

This is a good place to start to separate fact from fiction. It is easy to fall into the trap of, "Well, if so and so said it, it has to be true." Not everything you read or hear has 100% truth to it. As a fitness professional, I have fallen into the trap of fact versus fiction. I had to find out on my own. Let's take a look at 10 fitness myths and truths.

Myth #1: *Cardio and more Cardio is the only way to lose weight fast.*

FACT: Cardio alone burns away *both* fat and muscle. For a greater benefit, you have to incorporate strength training into your routine. Weight training build lean muscle mass; which increases your metabolism, and helps you burn more fat, even after exercise.

Myth #2: *If I exercise, I can eat whatever I want.*

FACT: Sure, you can eat whatever you want, but will it help you reach your goals? Calories in versus calories out are a key component to weight loss, but eating healthy will increase your likelihood of losing weight. While it is okay to have your favorite unhealthy foods, making it an everyday habit isn't productive. Think twice about that fast food burger after your hard earned workout. You can't exercise out a bad diet!

Myth #3: *I don't want to lift weights because I will get bulky.*

FACT: This one is for the ladies. You are doing yourself a disservice if you aren't weight training. As stated in the fact of the first myth, your body burns fat and increases your metabolism when weights are involved. Unless you are taking testosterone or steroids and lifting an excessive amount of weight, you will never get bulky, or look like a man. So, lift away!

Myth #4: *Doing crunches or working on an "ab machine" will get rid of belly fat.*

FACT: My favorite saying is, "Abs are made in the kitchen." This is so true! You can do all the sit ups in the world, but if your diet isn't up to par, you will never see those ab muscles. Not everyone expects the "Six Pack" abs, but losing the unsightly belly fat is top on almost everyone's fitness list. I get asked all the time what exercises will help the belly fat go away, and my answer every time is, "Diet"; plain and simple.

Myth #5: *Carbohydrates will make you fat.*

FACT: The role of carbohydrates in the body includes providing energy for working muscles and function of the body's organs. Carbohydrates should be your main source of fuel. However, processed foods, such as white bread, white rice, and pasta in excess, will increase your chances of gaining weight. Choosing healthy options such as fruits and vegetables and whole grains, will give you a greater benefit. I will go into further detail in the next chapter about carbohydrates.

Myth #6: *If I eat less, I will lose weight.*

FACT: Your body needs the fuel from food to function properly. You can reduce your caloric intake, but if it is too drastic, you could be doing more harm than good. Your body can go into "starvation" mode and to protect itself, begins to store fat. Know your body and make healthy food choices rather than try to go on an extremely low calorie diet, thinking this is the answer to weight loss.

Myth #7: *If I am not sore after my workout, I didn't do enough.*

FACT: Without going into too much detail and further confusing you, the soreness post exercise, or even a couple of days after; also referred to as *delayed onset muscle soreness* (DOMS), happens when you put your muscles under stress it isn't accustomed to. Just because you aren't sore doesn't mean you didn't work the muscles. There is lack of evidence that muscle soreness means a more effective workout.

Myth #8: *The scale determines my progress.*

FACT: Too many people get discouraged when they have been exercising and don't see the numbers changing on the scale. As a fitness professional, I constantly remind my clients that what they see on the scale shouldn't be their main focus.

 I had a previous client getting frustrated that his weight wasn't budging when he weighed himself, but informed me he had lost 6 inches around his waist in a matter of a couple of months. I was ecstatic. That is great! He was also lifting weights 4 days a week, increasing the weight as he progressed. While his weight didn't change much, he was losing inches and his clothing was probably fitting better than before.

In the End

While there are truths and myths to everything, sometimes you need to find out the truths for yourself. It can be easy to say, "If they said I shouldn't do it, I just won't do it". 30 years ago we didn't have the social media sources we have today. So much is circulating on the internet that it is hard to discern from what is true or false.

Understand Training Variables

Before designing your exercises, it is important to understand the variables associated with exercise; how many repetitions to do, sets, rest, training frequency, including duration.

Repetitions

Repetition is a thing repeated. In the case of exercise, it would be a complete movement of a particular exercise. Repetitions are simply a way to count the number of movements performed in a given amount of time. Let's say you are doing squats. Your goal is to repeat the movement 10 times, therefore 10 repetitions.

Sets

A set is a group of continuous repetitions. So you have determined you want to do 10 squats continuous 3 times. You would be performing 3 sets. Example: 10 repetitions of squats for 3 sets.

Rest Interval

The rest interval is the time taken to recuperate from an exercise before continuing on. Depending on your fitness level, your rest interval will be anywhere from 0 seconds to 3 minutes. Each exercise that is performed requires energy. The longer your rest interval, you allow your muscles to recover and regain energy to continue with the current exercise.

Training Frequency

The training frequency refers to the amount of training sessions during a period of time (typically in 1 week). The number of training sessions per week is determined by several factors, including your training goals, general health, age, how quickly you recover, and work capacity.

Training Duration

Training duration has 2 prominent meanings: The timeframe from the start of your workout to the end, and the length of time spent in one particular period of training (beginner exercises to intermediate to advanced, etc.).

Exercise Selection

This is the process of choosing exercises that accommodate to your needs and wants to achieve the desired results. When you have certain conditions (knee replacement, shoulder injuries, high blood pressure, diabetes), understanding what exercises you can and cannot do are vital. Always consult with your doctor if you have special conditions that would create difficulties of certain exercises.

Now you should have a clear understanding of how to design your fitness program. Let's move on to how to set up your workout regimen using a weekly plan.

Sample Weekly Plan

Table 5.1 is an example of a weekly plan to exercise. This is a beginner regimen for those who are exercising at home.

Table 5.1

Weekly Workout at Home: Beginners

Monday: Cardio
Goal: 45 minutes of jogging

Tuesday: Body Weight Training
Goal: 30 minutes of exercise
Exercises: Jumping Jacks, Squats, Mountain Climbers, High Knees, Butt Kicks, Lunges.
10 Repetitions, 4 Sets, 30 second to 1 minute rest between sets.

Wednesday: Rest

Thursday: Intense Cardio
Goal: 1 hour of running outdoors

Friday: Body Weight Training
Goal: 45 minutes of exercise
Exercises: Plank hold 30 seconds, Crunches, Mountain Climbers, Jump Rope, Side Plank hold 30 seconds each side, Lunges, Step ups, Squat Jumps.
12 Repetitions, 4 sets, 30 second to 1 minute rest between sets.

Saturday and Sunday can be rest or light cardio.

Sample Weekly Plan

Table 5.2 is an example of a weekly plan if you are working out at a gym. This is a sample beginner plan.

Table 5.2
Weekly Workout at the Gym: Beginners

Monday: Cardio
Goal: 30 minutes jogging on the treadmill, 15 minutes elliptical

Tuesday: Weight Training
Goal: 30 minutes of exercise
Exercises: Chest press, seated row, overhead shoulder press, bicep curls, triceps press down, leg press, calf raises.
10 Repetitions, 3 Sets, 30 second to 1 minute rest between sets.

Wednesday: Rest

Thursday: Intense Cardio
Goal: 45 mins run and walk on treadmill-1 min slow, 1.5 min fast

Friday: Weight Training
Goal: 45 minutes of exercise
Exercises: Crunch machine, cable fly, pulldown, upright row kettlebell, dumbbell bicep curl, triceps kickback, leg extension, hamstring curl, squats on the bosu.
12 Repetitions, 3 sets, 30 second to 1 minute rest between sets.

Saturday and Sunday can be rest or light cardio.

Dumbbells, kettlebells, barbells, oh my!

Whether you choose to workout at home or at a gym, getting a grasp on all the names of the equipment can be a daunting task. As a beginner myself at one time, I knew the basics. Over the years, the selection of equipment has multiplied. It can be intimidating to go to a gym and not know what everything does. You're afraid of looking stupid because you are doing it all wrong. As you progress month by month, you might want to change up your routine as you grow out of beginner status.

Fitness should be exciting and new, not boring. I want to give you a definition of the typical exercise equipment you may see in the gym or when you are searching for home equipment online or in stores:

Dumbbells: By definition is a short bar with a weight at each end; aka free weight, is a weight that can be used individually or in both hands. Ranges in weight are from 1 pound to over 100 pounds.

Exercises using dumbbells: Bicep curl, bent over row, triceps overhead press, shoulder press, squats, standing calf raises, to name a few.

Kettlebells: Kettlebells were developed in Russia. Unlike traditional dumbbells, kettlebells are designed for "swinging" movements. The description of a kettlebell is a round weight with a flat bottom and a thick handle on top. Kettlebells weight varies and can be measured in Kilograms or Pounds.

Exercises using kettlebells: Kettlebell swing, renegade row, upright row, Russian twist, goblet squat

Barbells: A long metal bar to which disks of varying weights are attached at each end. Typically gyms will have barbells that are labeled with the size at the end of the weight that isn't detachable. Sizes vary from 20 pounds to 100 pounds, usually.

Exercises using barbells: chest press, close grip press, upright row, bent over row, bicep curls, front or back squats.

Medicine Ball: A heavy, solid, round ball used typically for catching and throwing exercises. Medicine balls usually come in sizes 2-25 pounds.

Exercises using a medicine ball: Russian twist, lift and chop, overhead triceps press, lunge to twist, rolling push up, wall throw, and shoulder press.

Bosu Ball: The name is an acronym meaning, "Both Sides Up." A bosu has one side that is flat made of plastic with handles, and the other side is a rubber hemisphere mainly used for balance exercises.

Exercises using a bosu ball: Single leg balance, squats, push-ups, forearm plank, and a glute bridge.

Resistance Bands: An elastic band with handles at each end and resembles a jump rope. Sizes are defined by the color of the band. Typically yellow (3-5 pounds of resistance) to black (15-20 pounds). Each manufacturer may use a different color system.

Exercises using resistance bands: Bicep curl, triceps extension, front raises, lateral side walk, seated row.

TRX- Most gyms today have a TRX suspension system, which is a **T**otal-body **R**esistance e**x**ercise. You use your own body weight to perform the exercises in either a horizontal or even vertical fashion.

Exercises using the TRX Suspension trainer: Chest press, row, shoulder raises, bicep curl, triceps overhead, squats, suspended crunches (knee ins).

Machines: Machines at gym will vary. Exercise machines at a gym will keep you in a fixed position, which are great for beginner's who are unsure of their form. As you progress from beginner to intermediate, you will find yourself using the machines less and less. A benefit of using a machine as a novice is they are usually labeled what they are and what muscles are being used. Here are some examples of machines you may see at a gym:

Seated incline chest press, lat pull down, bicep curl, triceps extension, shoulder press, leg extension, abdominal crunch, just to name a few.

Now that you have a clearer picture of the typical pieces of equipment used in a gym, let's design a beginner's workout using these items.

Table 5.3 is a beginner's workout for a single session. This session is about an hour in length. Starting out, use a lighter weight.

Table 5.3

Sample Single Session Workout at the Gym

Warm Up- Treadmill 5 minutes

Exercise #1- Incline Chest Press (machine) 10 reps x 3 sets
Exercise #2- Bench Press (barbell) 10 reps x 3 sets
Exercise #3- Bent over row (dumbbells) 10 reps x 3 sets
Exercise #4- Lat pull down (machine) 10 reps x 3 sets
Exercise #5- Kettlebell upright row 10 reps x 3 sets
Exercise #6- Lateral raises (dumbbells) 10 reps x 3 sets
Exercise #7- Bicep curl (dumbbells) 10 reps x 3 sets
Exercise #8- Concentration curl (dumbbells) 10 reps x 3 sets
Exercise #9- Triceps extension (machine) 10 reps x 3 sets
Exercise #10- triceps overhead (dumbbells) 10 reps x 3 sets
Exercise #11- Leg press (machine) 10 reps x 3 sets
Exercise #12- Kettlebell swing 10 reps x 3 sets
Exercise #13- Russian twist (medicine ball) 10 reps x 3 sets
Exercise #14- Abdominal crunch (machine) 10 reps x 3 sets

Cool down- 30 second stretch, each body part. Treadmill or exercise bike for 10 minutes at a slow pace.

The Do's and Don'ts of Weight Training

You might learn training techniques by watching friends or others at a gym, but what you see may not always be correct or even safe. Incorrect weight training technique can lead to sprains, strains, fractures, and other painful injuries that may hinder your weight training efforts.

If you are just getting started, it might be wise to work with a knowledgeable weight training specialist (aka certified personal trainer) who is familiar with proper form and technique. I will go over the do's and don'ts of lifting to get you going.

Lifting Do's

Lift and appropriate amount of weight: Start with a weight you can comfortably lift without strain for 10-12 times. As you get stronger, you will gradually increase the amount of weight.

Breathe: It can be tempting to hold your breath when you are lifting weights. Holding your breath can lead to an increase in blood pressure. Be sure to exhale as you lift the weight.

Use proper form: The better your form, the better the results and the less likely you are to injure yourself. If you are unable to maintain proper form, decrease your weight. I will further discuss proper form in the next section.

Rest: Avoid exercising the same muscles two days in a row. The rest allows the muscles to rebuild and repair. 48

hours or 2 days between working the same muscles is crucial. The downside of not resting the muscles is a higher risk of overtraining. Extreme fatigue and weakness can be a sign.

Lifting Don'ts

Don't rush through the workout: Moving the weight in a hurried fashion could lead to injury and little results. Taking it slow helps you isolate the muscles you want to work and keeps you from relying on momentum to lift the weight. Unless your goal is endurance, lifting the weights in a fast motion won't you much good.

Don't skip the warm up: Cold muscles are more prone to injury than warm muscles. Before you weight train, warm up for at least 5 minutes with brisk walking or a dynamic warm up, moving all body parts.

Don't ignore pain: If an exercise causes pain, stop. Try it again after a few days with a lower weight.

Don't overdo it: As a beginner, it is easy to fall in the trap of wanting to do more than you should, trying to reach your goal faster. This can lead to injury and lack a motivation, especially when you become fatigued at every workout.

There are no quick fixes

As with most things in life, we are in a hurry to get to the next step as quick as possible. In fitness, I always see people wanting to get to their goal quickly, but not understanding that it takes time. You didn't pack on 30 pounds overnight and you will not lose the weight overnight either. See each new day as new beginning, a fresh start to make it right.

As we move forward, I will be giving examples of exercises I see people doing incorrectly all the time. Learning proper form is vital.

Flat Bench Chest Press

Beginners can start out using the Smith Machine for the chest press if they are uncomfortable using a barbell. The smith machine is in a fixed position and has "stoppers" so if you lose your grip, the bar will not come crashing down on you. First choose an appropriate weight to start out with. As you lay your back on the bench, make sure the bar is at the upper chest level. Your hands will be at least shoulder width apart (if you have shoulder concerns, shoulder width or just inside shoulder width is recommended to avoid injury or pain), keep your wrists in neutral position (avoid bending the wrist when performing the exercise. Slowly lower the bar to the chest and press back up. If you notice your back starts to arch, you are compensating and may need to lower the weight or take longer rest periods between sets.

Bent over Barbell Row

Choose your weight. This is a standing exercise. Grip the barbell with palms facing down, hinge slightly forward from your hips, keeping your back straight (use the mirror at the gym to see yourself) bring the barbell into your ribs, squeezing your shoulder blades together, then slowly lower back so the arms are straight down.

Pull Downs

This is the most common exercise I see people doing incorrectly. While every person may tell you different, pulling the bar behind your neck can cause injury, strain to the neck, and defeat the purpose of the entire exercise. Pull down machines have an adjustable weight, so choose the weight you want first. Grab the bar handle to should width or closer in, for a normal pull down, grip the bar palms down, pull bar to your chest, having a slight lean back then slowly release bar back up.

Dumbbell Shoulder Lateral Raises

Pick same weight dumbbells that will be appropriate for you to lift to the shoulders. You can perform this exercise seated or standing. Keeping neutral wrist position, raise arms to your sides, keeping your arms straight. If you have shoulder concerns, do not raise the dumbbells up higher than your shoulders. Lower weight back down in a slow, controlled manner.

Standing Dumbbell Bicep Curls

If you are new to exercise, it may be better to start with single arm dumbbell bicep curls to help control the weight versus two arms, where you may have a tendency to swing the arms. Choose your weight, keep your upper arm in a locked position (do not move your upper arm the entire exercise), hinging from the elbow bring arm up to about chest level with neutral wrists and slowly lower back to start. The moment you begin to twist your wrists in towards your body, you are now compensating and not performing the exercise to its full potential.

Triceps Kickback using Dumbbells

This exercise can be done standing or kneeling on a bench. Beginners I typically start standing. You will use one weight at a time, so pick the weight you want to use. With the dumbbell in one hand, place the other hand on the wall and bring the leg back that has the dumbbell in your hand, bending the opposite knee, bringing your arm parallel with the extended leg back. Keeping your upper arm isolated, start by bringing your lower arm in (only hinging from the elbow) and extending it straight back, wrists in neutral position. I always see people wanting to twist the wrist back as they bring the arm back, but again, this is a common compensation, and the weight is too heavy. Lower the weight as needed.

Squats (back squat)

Whether you want to do body or weighted squats using a barbell, proper technique is required. If you have never done a squat, you can safely start with a wall ball squat. Grab a stability ball ,place it on the wall and squat to your comfort, feet are shoulder width apart and knees should not go over your toes, this can cause discomfort in the knee should you go past the toes. Without assistance from a stability ball, pretend you are going to sit down into a chair. You would put your butt back first, and avoid rounding or arching the back as you descend back. For body weight, you can bring your arms in front of you for stability. For the weighed squat, place the barbell at your upper back, avoiding contact with your spine. If you squeeze your shoulder blades in, you have a cushion to place the barbell on. Keeping feet shoulder width apart, you will hip hinge back as if you are sitting in a chair. Again, keep your eyes facing forward as you descend down.

Stiff Leg Deadlift

This is top on my list of the exercise most commonly performed incorrectly. This exercise when performed correctly focuses on improving your hamstrings, glutes, and back, so it is a great exercise and one of my personal favorites. You will use a barbell to do this exercise. Feet shoulder width apart, starting in an upright position with the back nice and straight, hip hinge forward, keeping the barbell close to the body, legs are almost straight, but with a slight bend, lower the barbell to the center of the shins or to the toes. Keep the natural curvature in the back but try to avoid excessive rounding (you may need to lower the weight); you want to bring the barbell back to neutral, hinging back up from the hip to a straight position.

While there are so many different exercises out there, I have outlined a few, maybe the most common exercises I see on a daily basis. As you progress in this process, you will find what works for you and what doesn't. You will find exercises you enjoy and exercise you loathe. It's a learning experience.

Chapter 7

Nutrition Basics

We live in a world of a rapidly changing environment. To accommodate to our "busy" lifestyle, our food supply has made it easier for us to eat on the go. Food quality is not the same as it was 30 years ago. More and more people are looking for a quick meal, and not necessarily a healthy one. This has led to the obesity epidemic the United States is now facing. Nearly 1/3 of U.S. adults are obese. In this chapter, you will learn the basic nutrients needed for health and provide you with helpful hints to be successful in your health and fitness journey.

What is Nutrition?

By definition, nutrition is the process of providing or obtaining the food necessary for health and growth. Food is a necessity of life. More broadly, nutrition is the science of food and determining what nutrients are required. This science determines how your body ingests, digests, absorbs, metabolizes, transports, and stores different foods. The four essential nutrients that will be discussed in the chapter are: carbohydrates, fats, proteins, and water.

Carbohydrates

Carbohydrates are the most important source of fuel in supplying energy to your body. Carbohydrates provide the body with glucose, which is converted into energy used to support bodily function and physical activity.

Many people are confused about carbohydrates, not truly understanding that carbohydrates are essential. It is more important to eat carbohydrates from healthy foods than follow a strict diet limiting the grams of carbohydrates consumed.

What are Carbohydrates?

Carbohydrates are made up of carbon, hydrogen, and oxygen and generally classified as simple (sugars), complex (starches), and fiber.

Carbohydrates are found in both healthy and unhealthy foods such as bread, beans, pasta, rice, corn, cookies, nuts, and soda, just to name a few.

Foods high in carbohydrates are important part of a healthy diet. According to the Dietary Reference Intakes published by the USDA, carbohydrates should account for 45% to 65% of your daily intake. Complex carbohydrates (whole grains, fruits and vegetables) should constitute for the majority of your calories.

Carbohydrates also help regulate fat and metabolize protein. Each gram of carbohydrate provides 4 calories.

Simple Carbohydrates

Simple carbohydrates are called simple sugars. Sugars are found in a variety of natural food sources including fruit, vegetables, and milk, but are also found in processed foods like candy, soda, syrup, and cake.

Simple carbohydrates are broken down quickly by the body to be used as energy. All simple carbohydrates are made up of either one or two sugar molecules; Monosaccharides, which include glucose, fructose and galactose and disaccharides, which include sucrose, lactose, and maltose.

Here are some common foods that contain high levels of simple carbohydrates:

1. **Soft Drinks** – Many non-diet soft drinks (soda or pop) are loaded with sugar. Coca Cola's 12 fl oz. can of soda has 39 grams of sugar, with the ingredient label reading high **fructose** corn syrup as its second ingredient.

2. **Fruit Juices** – Many people think that because juice is made of fruit, it is healthy for you. Fruit juices contain a large amount of simple carbohydrates (sugar). Typical apple juice contains 24 grams of sugar in an 8 fl oz. drink.

3. **Yogurt** - While there are healthier options for yogurt, most contain a high amount of sugar. Growing up, Yoplait was popular. I reviewed the label for Yoplait's Original Cherry and the second ingredient is sugar, containing 26 grams of sugar and 33 grams of carbohydrates in a 6 oz. container.

4. **Fruit Snacks** – Just because it has "fruit" in the name doesn't mean it is good for you! Fruit snacks are a processed food containing a high amount a sugar. The main ingredients in Kellogg's fruit snacks are Corn Syrup and Sugar!

It can be really easy to think you are eating healthy when "fruit" is in the title of a product. The best choice would be eating the fruit itself. Below you will find a short list of simple carbohydrates that are good for you, in moderation of course!

- Bananas
- Blueberries
- Apples
- Strawberries
- Oranges
- Cherries
- Pears

For those times you crave something sweet, reach for that banana instead of fruit snacks or that candy bar. Fruits are a great source of vitamins that help protect your body against disease.

So, at your next trip to the grocery store, think about adding those fruits to your shopping cart. Your body will thank you!

Complex Carbohydrates

Complex carbohydrates, unlike simple carbohydrates contain three or more sugar molecules (polysaccharides) including starch, fiber, and glycogen. Complex carbohydrates digest in the body slowly, delivering a steady supply of sugar (energy) to the body. The fiber content in complex carbohydrates also aids in satiety (that feeling of being satisfied or full), so you can resist eating more than you need.

Complex carbohydrates provide vitamins, minerals, and fiber that are important to the health of an individual. The majority of carbohydrates should come from these complex carbohydrates (starches) and naturally occurring sugars, rather than processed or refined sugars, which provide little to no nutritional value.

"Healthy Carbs"

Healthy carbs are those that are in their natural state or whole, and require little to no processing. Examples of healthy carbs are your leafy green vegetables, whole grains (brown rice, quinoa, and whole wheat), starchy vegetables such as sweet potatoes and corn, nuts (almonds, sunflower seeds, pistachios, and peanuts) Beans (lentils, black beans, kidney beans, and pinto beans).

While this is not a complete list, you can see the types of complex carbohydrates that are healthy for you. Hopefully you have a better understanding of carbohydrates and will be able to choose healthier options.

Fats

Many foods contain several different types of fat, and some are better for your health than others. Some fats actually help promote good health. The fats you eat give your body energy that is needs to work properly. Fat also helps absorb vitamins A, D, E, and K.

Fat has 9 calories per gram and should be the lowest percentage in your diet consisting of approximately 20-35%.

Saturated Fats

Saturated fats are common in the American diet. Saturated fats are normally solid at room temperature. Most come from animal sources such as beef, poultry, whole-fat milk, cheese and butter, even coconut oil.

A diet rich in saturated fats can raise the level LDL cholesterol (aka: bad cholesterol). Foods that contain trans-fat (partially hydrogenated oil) are the worst type of fat.

Research from the Harvard School of Public Health indicates that trans-fats can harm health even in small amounts: for every 2% of calories from trans-fat consumed daily, the risk of heart disease increases by 23%.

Unsaturated Fats

Unsaturated fats are the healthier or "good" fats. Unsaturated fats come primarily from plant foods, such as nuts and seeds, and are liquid at room temperature. Examples include vegetable oils such as olive, peanut, safflower, and sunflower. Unlike saturated fats, unsaturated fats do not raise blood cholesterol. Unsaturated fats are either monounsaturated or polyunsaturated or a combination of both. Monounsaturated fats aid in reducing high blood cholesterol and raise the HDL, or "good" cholesterol.

Good sources of monounsaturated fats are olive oil, peanut oil, canola oil, avocados, and most nuts.

Here are some tips to help you choose healthy fat in your diet:

- Read labels. This topic will be further discussed in the next chapter, but be aware of the fats in the products you choose.
- Use liquid vegetable oil instead of solid fats. For example, used olive oil instead of butter when sautéing vegetables.
- Use olive oil in salad dressings and marinades.
- Choose egg whites over whole eggs when possible.
- Bake or broil instead of frying, especially deep frying.

It is always best to do as much research as possible to completely understand what is "good" and "bad" for you.

I have provided a general breakdown to help you understand in an easier way.

Proteins

Proteins are long chain molecules built from small units known as amino acids. They are joined together by peptide bonds.

Protein is referred to as the building block of the body. Protein is vital in the maintenance and repair of body tissue.

There are 20 common amino acids that are vital to life and health. They are categorized as essential, non-essential, and semi-essential. Essential amino acids cannot be manufactured by the body; they must be obtained through food supply. Non-essential (as you may have guessed) amino acids can be manufactured by the body. Semi- essential amino acids are normally considered non-essential amino acids because the body can make them; however, under circumstances such as illness, the body cannot make them at high enough levels, and they become an essential amino acid.

Food Sources of Protein

According to the United States Department of Agriculture, all food made from meat, poultry, seafood, beans and peas, eggs, nut and seeds are considered part of the protein group.

Choose a variety of protein foods to improve health benefits; this is also the key to a balanced diet. Food proteins are classified as complete and incomplete, depending on their amino acid composition.

Complete Proteins

A complete protein is a protein that contains all of the essential amino acids. These proteins are primarily of animal origin (meat, poultry, fish, egg, milk, and cheese). However, soy products are the only plant sources of complete proteins; good news for those who are vegetarian.

Incomplete Proteins

Incomplete protein is any protein that is lacking one or more of the essential amino acids. These proteins are generally of plant origin (grains, legumes, seeds, and nuts).

Too much protein

The Recommended Dietary Allowances (RDA) suggests that 10-35% should be the obtained about for your total caloric intake of protein.

Eating excess protein does not build muscle; only exercising with enough protein to support growth can do that. High protein diets can have excess amounts of saturated fat, potentially leading to cardiovascular disease. If you eat more protein than your body requires, it will simply convert most of those calories to sugar and then to fat. The more physically active you are, the more protein you will ingest. As a fitness professional and enthusiast, typically 1 gram per pound of body weight of protein is suggested.

Just like with your carbohydrates and fats, calories in versus calories out will ultimately lead to weight loss. Everyone responds differently to foods, so listen to your body first and foremost.

The information provided regarding carbohydrates, fats, and proteins are suggestions only. Consult with your doctor if you have certain conditions or diseases before seeking a change in your diet.

Water

Water is a colorless, transparent, odorless, and tasteless liquid.

Your body makes up 60% of your body weight. Every system in your body depends on water. As an example, water flushes toxins out of vital organs, and carries nutrients to your cells.

Lack of water can lead to dehydration, a condition that occurs when you do not have enough water in your body to carry out normal functions.

How much water do I need?

You may have heard the advice, "Drink eight 8-ounce glasses of water a day." While that is not supported by conclusive evidence, it remains popular because it is easy to remember. Everybody is different; if you are an athlete, such as a runner or sprinter, you will require more water to replenish what your body has lost during exercise. Relatively speaking, if you are a sedentary male, your water consumption per day should be around 13 cups. For a sedentary female, it is suggested to consume approximately 9 cups. Water consumption should also be increased for those residing in a dry, hot climate.

Dehydration

Dehydration occurs when your use or lose more fluid than you take in, and your body doesn't have enough water and other fluids to provide normal function to your body.

Common causes of dehydration include intense exercise, excessive sweating, not drinking enough water every day, and when you have the flu; with vomiting and diarrhea. Excess alcohol consumption can also lead to dehydration (and a pounding headache!) You can usually reverse mild to moderate dehydration by drinking more fluids, but severe dehydration needs medical attention.

Signs of Dehydration

Mild to moderate dehydration:

- Dry mouth
- Sleepiness or feeling tired
- Thirst
- Headache
- Dizziness
- Constipation

- Dry Skin

Severe dehydration:

- Extreme thirst
- Little or no urination
- Sunken eyes
- Rapid breathing
- Rapid heart beat
- Fever
- In most serious cases, delirium or unconsciousness.

While thirst isn't always a reliable measure to determine the body's need for water, the color of your urine is a better indicator. Clear or light-colored urine means you are well hydrated, whereas a dark yellow or amber color usually signals dehydration.

Prevention

To prevent dehydration, drink plenty of fluids and eat foods with a high water content such as fruits and vegetables.

Drink plenty of water before, during, and after you are active; if you are exercising for more than an hour, you may want to consider a sports drink that contains electrolytes, to restore balance in the body.

Summary

Consuming an adequate amount of water will help regulate body temperature, rids the body of toxins, lubricates your joints, it can even aid in controlling calories (drinking water and eat water-rich foods that are dense will help you feel full quicker, reducing the amount you eat each day).

The importance of proper hydration cannot be stressed enough. Our bodies cannot adapt to dehydration, which impairs every anatomical function. The human body can only survive without water for a few days.

Finally, there is no more important nutrient for our bodies than water. All humans need water to survive. Water keeps you healthy and alive!

Chapter 8

Healthy Eating

What is healthy eating? Healthy eating means eating a variety of foods that provide you with the nutrients your body needs to sustain good health.

Eating healthy can help reduce the risk of diabetes, high blood pressure, certain types of cancer, and helps in maintaining a healthy weight. According to the *Dietary Guidelines for Americans*, eating healthy means consuming a variety of nutritious foods and beverages including; vegetables, fruits, whole grains and low fat dairy products; limiting the intake of saturated fat, added sugars, and sodium.

In this chapter you will learn about the basic food groups, the importance of choosing the right foods, and dietary balance. We will start with the basic food groups.

What are the basic food groups?

This section will help explain the basic food groups based on the *Dietary Guidelines for Americans, 2010*. There are five food groups consisting of vegetables, fruits, grains, dairy, and a protein group that includes meat, poultry, fish, and nuts. *MyPlate* illustrates these five food groups that are essential for a healthy diet using a place setting for a meal to display how much of each food group you need to eat healthy. In table 8.1 you will see the ChooseMyPlate.Gov image first introduced 2011, to aid in building a healthy meal.

TABLE 8.1

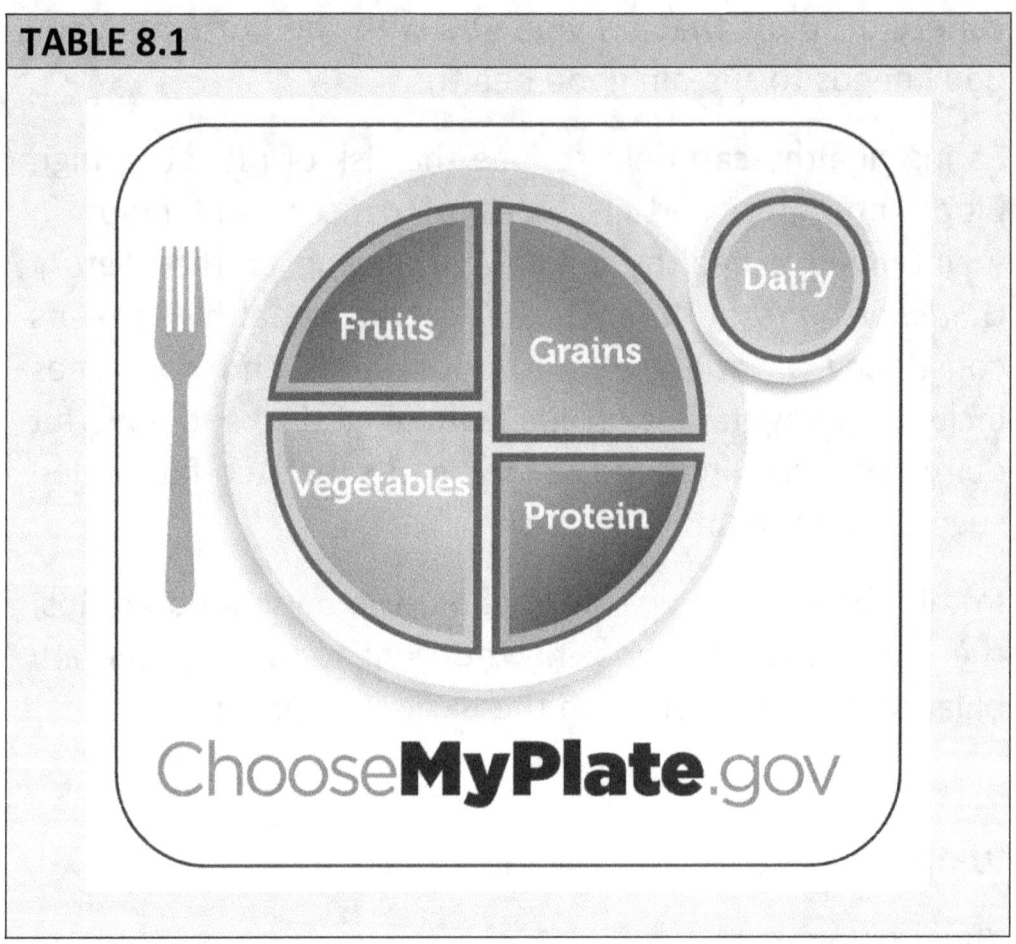

Vegetables

The vegetables you can eat may be fresh, frozen, canned or dried and may be eaten whole, cut up, or mashed. It is recommended that you eat a variety of dark green, red and orange vegetables, as well as beans and peas.

Examples include broccoli, carrots, collard greens, green beans, black-eyed peas, potatoes, lima beans, squash, sweet potatoes, tomatoes and kidney beans. Any vegetable or 100% vegetable juice is included in this group.

How much is needed for healthy eating?

The amount of vegetables varies for the needs of every individual based on age, level of activity, and gender. Typically women between the ages of 19-50 are recommended to eat two and a half cups a day of vegetables, men 19-50 about three cups per day.

What is the importance of eating vegetables?

Vegetables are importance sources of many nutrients including potassium, fiber, folic acid, vitamin A, and vitamin C.

Diets rich in potassium may help maintain healthy blood pressure. Vegetable sources of potassium include sweet potatoes, soybeans, lentils, tomato products (paste, sauce, and juice), and kidney beans.

Fiber from vegetables could help reduce blood cholesterol levels and may lower the risk of heart disease. Fiber is important for proper bowel function and helps with constipation. Fiber rich foods also help provide a feeling of fullness with fewer calories. Beans contain fiber.

Folic Acid helps the body form red blood cells. Consuming the right amount of folic acid before and during pregnancy helps prevent certain birth defects, including spina bifida. Folate occurs naturally in dark leafy green vegetables, legumes, and citrus fruits and juices.

Vitamin A keeps the eyes and skin healthy and helps protect against infection. Vegetable food sources include carrots, sweet potatoes, and bell peppers.

Vitamin C helps heal cuts and wounds, it also keeps teeth and gums healthy. Vitamin C aids in iron absorption. Vegetables high in vitamin C include yellow bell peppers, kale, broccoli, and spinach.

Eating vegetables provides health benefits. Those who consume more vegetables as part of their overall healthy diet are likely to have a reduced risk of some chronic diseases. Vegetables provide nutrients vital for health and maintenance of your body.

Fruits

The fruits you eat may be fresh, canned, frozen, or dried and could be eaten whole, cut-up, or pureed. Examples include apples, bananas, grapes, dates, apricots, oranges, grapefruit, mangos, melons, peaches, pineapples, raisins, strawberries, tangerines, and 100% fruit juice.

How much fruit is needed for healthy eating?

The same rule that applies to vegetables also applies to fruit consumption. Typically both men and women ages 19-30 are recommended to consume two cups of fruit per day. Half of your plate should now be made up of vegetables and fruit. It is not saying you should eat fruit with every meal, but the entire daily consumption of fruit may equate to two cups. For example, you may eat a banana as your mid-morning snack. The banana would equal one cup of the two cups recommended for the day.

Why is it important to eat fruit?

Most fruits are low in calories and fat and are a source of simple sugars, fiber, and can provide antioxidants that are needed for good health. Eating fruit as a snack is a great way to satisfy your sweet tooth and get the extra nutrition you want. Eating foods such as fruits that are lower in calories per cup instead of some other higher calorie foods may help aid in a lower calorie intake.

Helpful tips

In general, keep a bowl of fruit out on the table, counter, or in the refrigerator. Buy fresh fruits when they are in season, as they may be less expensive and at their peak flavor. Refrigerate cut-up fruits to keep for later.

To make the most of your fruit choices, pick whole or cut-up fruit rather than juice for the most benefits. When choosing canned fruits, select fruit canned in 100% fruit juice or water rather than heavy syrup. The last and most important tip in fruit is to always rinse fruits before preparing or eating them.

Remember, fruit is healthy and delicious. Eating fruits provide health benefits- those who eat more fruits as part of their overall diet are likely to reduce the risk of certain diseases. Fruits as with vegetables provide the nutrients necessary for the health and maintenance of your body.

Grains

There are two types of grains – whole and refined grains. At least half of the grains you eat should be whole grains; whole-wheat bread, oatmeal, bulgur, and brown rice. Refined grains include white bread, white rice, enriched pasta, tortillas, and most noodles.

How many grain foods are needed daily?

The amount of grains you need depends on your age, gender, and level of physical activity. Most Americans consume enough grains, but not enough whole grains. At least half of all grains eaten should be whole grains. The total daily recommended serving of grains for women age 19-50 is equivalent to six ounces, of which 3 ounces should be whole grains. For men age 19-50 is 8 ounces (7 ounces for 31-50), of which 4 ounces would be whole grains.

The importance of grains, especially whole grains

Grains are an importance source of many nutrients including fiber, vitamins (thiamin, riboflavin, niacin, and folate), and minerals (magnesium, iron, and selenium).

The B vitamins thiamin, riboflavin, and niacin help the body release energy from protein, fat, and carbohydrates; and play a key role in metabolism.

Whole grains are a good source of magnesium and selenium. Magnesium is a key mineral in building bones and releasing energy from muscles. Selenium has antioxidant components that may help protect cells from damage.

Iron is used to carry oxygen in the blood. Your body needs the right amount of iron. If you have too little iron, you may develop the iron deficiency, anemia. Iron-fortified breakfast cereals have a higher content of iron than most foods.

Eat more whole grains

To eat more whole grains, substitute a whole-grain food in place of a refined food – such as eating brown rice instead of white rice and whole-grain bread instead of white bread.

Below is a list of food items that are whole grain:

- Whole wheat
- Brown rice
- Quinoa
- Corn

- Steel cut oats
- Barley
- Buckwheat
- Bulgur (cracked wheat)
- Millet (whole grain flour)

What to look for on food labels

When shopping at the grocery store, it is important to read the label carefully, especially the ingredients. Foods labeled with the words "multi-grain", "100% wheat", "cracked wheat", "seven-grain", or "bran" are usually not whole grain products.

Read the food labels ingredients list. Look for words that indicate added sugars (such as sucrose, high-fructose corn syrup, malt syrup, molasses, or raw sugar), that add extra calories.

Most sodium in the food supply comes from packaged foods. Foods with less than 140 mg per serving can be labeled as low sodium foods.

So next time you visit your local food market, you will have a better understanding of what to look for in whole grain foods.

Dairy

The fourth basic food group we will be discussing is the dairy group. All fluid milk products and many foods made from milk are considered part of this food group. Most choices can be low-fat or fat-free, but all milks and calcium-containing milk products count in the category. Examples include milk, cheese, and yogurt as well as lactose-free products. Foods that are made from milk but have little or no calcium are not included, such as butter, cream, sour cream, and cream cheese.

How much dairy do I need?

The amount of food from the dairy group you need to eat depends on age. Typically after the age of eight years old, 3 cups are recommended.

Consuming dairy products provide health benefits, especially for bone health. Nutrients found in dairy products include calcium, potassium, vitamin D, and protein.

Nutrients

Calcium is important for building strong bones and teeth. Diets that provide 3 cups or the equivalent of dairy products per day can improve bone mass.

Diets high in potassium can help improve blood pressure. Dairy products such as yogurt, fluid milk, and soymilk, provide potassium.

Vitamin D is vital to strong bones and a healthy immune system. Vitamin D aids in the absorption of calcium and phosphorous. Milk and soymilk that are fortified with vitamin D are good sources of this nutrient.

Milk and milk products like cheese and yogurt are high in protein content. There are two types of protein found in milk products, casein and whey. Whey is quickly broken down into amino acids and absorbed into the bloodstream. Casein is digested more slowly and provides the body with a steady supply of protein for a longer period of time.

The Health Benefits

Intake of dairy products is linked to improved bone health, and may help reduce the risk of osteoporosis. Consuming dairy products during childhood and adolescence is especially important to build strong bones while they are still in the growing stages. Intake of dairy products is also associated with a reduced risk of cardiovascular disease, type 2 diabetes, and lowering blood pressure as well as maintaining a healthy weight.

Protein Foods

All foods made from meat, poultry, seafood, beans and peas, eggs, nuts and seeds are considered part of the protein food group. Select a variety of protein foods to improve nutrient intake and health benefits, including 8 ounces of cooked seafood a week (unless you are vegetarian) to help prevent heart disease.

How much protein do I need?

Just the same with all the other food groups, this is dependent upon your age, sex, and level of physical activity daily. Proteins from foods that are recommended are approximately five to six ounces a day, according to the US Department of Agriculture.

Keep it Lean

When choosing meat, start with a lean choice. The leanest beef cuts include top sirloin, top loin, round steaks and roasts (eye of round, top round, bottom round, round tip), and chuck shoulder.

Choose extra lean ground beef. The label should say at least "90% lean." You may be able to find ground beef that is even 93-95% lean.

Boneless skinless chicken breasts are the leanest poultry choices. Trim away any fat from poultry and meats before cooking.

Different Protein Choices

You can choose seafood at least twice a week as your main protein food. Look for seafood containing Omega-3 fatty acids, such as salmon, trout, and herring.

Consume beans, peas, or soy products as a main dish or part of a meal. A few choices are:

- Split pea, lentil, minestrone, or white bean soups
- Rice and beans
- Black bean enchiladas
- Veggie burgers
- Hummus (chickpeas) spread on pita bread

Choose unsalted nuts as a snack or on salads. Keep in mind, one serving of nuts is typically one-fourth of a cup. Read the food label to determine the amounts you want in eat.

Health Benefits

Meat, poultry, fish, beans and peas, eggs, nuts and seeds all supply many nutrients. These include protein, B vitamins (niacin, thiamin, riboflavin, and B6) vitamin E, iron, zinc, and magnesium.

Proteins function as building blocks for healthy bones, muscles, cartilage, skin, and blood. The body needs protein to repair itself. Adding protein to your diet is vital for the health and maintenance of your body.

A Balanced Diet

Now that you have learned about the basic food groups, it is important to understand why you should eat a balanced diet. To eat a balanced diet, you need to consume different types of foods from each of the main food groups.

A well-balanced diet can help your body fight many diseases and infections. When you consume enough of the vital nutrients, the immune system functions properly; this prevents infection and reduces the risk of chronic diseases like high blood pressure, diabetes, heart disease, and cancer.

Eating a balanced diet can also aid in maintaining a healthy weight. Choose foods that are low-fat or low calorie, and consume smaller portions.

Eating well is the key to maintaining a healthy immune system and preventing chronic diseases. The key to a healthy balanced diet is not to omit any foods or food groups, but to balance what you eat by consuming a variety of foods in the right proportions. The basic elements of a healthy diet include the right amount of carbohydrates, fat, protein, vitamins, minerals, and water.

Chapter 9

Meal Planning

"Those who fail to plan, plans to fail."

I bet a one time in your life you had your mind set to do something, but didn't follow through with it; it could be that you did not know how to plan or prepare.

In this chapter, you will learn the basics of how to plan and prepare for your meals, including shopping at the grocery store, how to read food labels, determine portion and serving sizes, and sample meal ideas.

Prepare for Success

As with any goal such as losing weight, exercising, or eating healthier, the first step is commitment. You should have a goal in mind and the steps it will take to accomplish that goal or goals. The same principle applies to meal planning:

- **Make a List**

Now that you know what foods are considered part of the food groups and are healthy for you, making a list either on paper or on your computer (to print out) of the meals you will make for the week. Start with meals you are familiar with that aren't too complicated to make.

- **Grocery Items List**

  In your first step, you planned out the meals you want to prepare and now you need to gather a list of items you will need for those meals. Look throughout your pantry and refrigerator to see what items you may already have, then compile a list of items you still need. You can write these items out on a piece of paper, or most handheld devices have apps that you are able to make a grocery list with (i.e. Out of Milk).

- **Set a Budget**

I have heard over and over again, "I can't afford healthy food". You would be surprised at how inexpensive eating healthy is compared to eating not so healthy. If you have several grocery stores located near your home, you can look to see which store has items on sale that you need. I personally never shop at just one store, but I live in a big city with many options. Not everyone can afford organic products, and that's okay. Set a food budget and get the items that you need for your meals.

At the Grocery Store

Now you have your list of items you need, and a set budget. First, do not go to the grocery store on an empty stomach! I have done this and it didn't end well. You may have a tendency to crave every food item possible. Everything looks good, and then you add items to your cart you do not need (or shouldn't be eating!).

Next, shop the outer sides of the grocery store first, since most of your food items should be located in these sections. The majority of stores will be laid out the same, fruits and vegetables either to the left or right of the store, and your meat and poultry items to the back or other side of the store; for the dairy products. The majority of processed foods are located in the middle, or aisles of the store.

Compare Name Brand to Store Brands

This can be quite the money saver! With many foods you wouldn't even know the difference in taste. Some store brands are even better than the name brands for much less. Some stores like Super Target even have coupons for their store brands. Also, read the food label to make sure they are comparable with the nutritional value.

Reading Food Labels

This is where I have found most people can get confused; how to read the food label. Food labels are on almost every food item in the supermarket (with the exception of fresh fruits and vegetables). The food label is either on the back or side of a food package. This label contains a variety of information about the nutritional value of the food item. On a standard food label you will find the serving size, the total amount of servings per package, the number of calories, grams of carbohydrates, fat, and protein, including other nutrients. This information helps people who are trying to limit their intake of fat, sodium sugar, or other ingredients, or those who are trying to get enough healthy nutrients such as vitamin C or calcium. The label provides each item with the approximate daily percent value, generally based on a 2,000 calorie diet. Below, you will see a typical nutrition facts label.

Nutrition Facts

Serving Size 1 cup (248g)

Serving Per Container 4

Amount Per Serving

Calories 150   Calories from Fat 70

% Daily Value *

Total Fat 8g	12%
Saturated Fat 4.0g	20%
Trans Fat 0g	
Cholesterol 20mg	7%
Sodium 170mg	7%
Total Carbohydrate 15g	10%
Dietary Fiber 0g	0%
Sugars 10g	
Protein 5g	
Vitamin A	4%
Vitamin C	6%
Calcium	40%
Iron	0%

*Percent Daily Values are based on a 2,000 calorie diet. Your Daily Values may be higher or lower depending on your calorie needs:

	Calories	2,000	2,500
Total Fat	Less Than	65g	80g
Sat Fat	Less Than	20g	25g
Cholesterol	Less Than	300mg	300mg
Sodium		Less Than	2,400mg
2,400mg			
Total Carbohydrate		300g	375g
Dietary Fiber		25g	30g

Calories per gram: Fat 9 Carbohydrates 4 Protein 4

Now let's decipher the food label:

Serving Size: The nutrition information applies to only one serving of food

Servings Per Container: The total amount in the container

Calories: The amount for one serving size. If you want to determine the total amount in the container, multiply the calories to the servings per container. Ex: 150 x 4 = 600 Calories

Total Fat: The total grams of fat in one serving of food. Avoid foods that are high in saturated fat and avoid trans-fat. Some food labels will also have listed *Polyunsaturated* and *Monounsaturated* fat, these are good for you.

Daily Value: Off to the right of the food label, you will see percentages of the nutrients in the product. These values are based on a 2,000 calorie diet. If you look at the bottom of the nutrition facts label, you will see the amount already calculated for a 2,000 and 2,500 calorie diet. For example, this label has 15g of carbohydrates, for a 2,000 calorie diet the amount of carbohydrates recommended is 300g daily. So the 15g carbohydrate value is only 10% of your daily carbohydrate intake.

Depending on your needs and goals, you might not need or use all the information on the nutrition facts label. You might be limiting your sugar intake and want foods that have less than 10 grams of sugar per serving. You need more fiber in your diet, so you look for items that have 5 or more grams a fiber per serving. Regardless of your goal, you should know what a serving size is and how many servings are in the container. By knowing this, you are able to interpret the information on the food label.

Portion Control

Now that you have a grasp on the how to read the food label, we can discuss how to portion out your meals for weight loss success. Portion size is very important if you are trying to lose weight and keep it off. We live in a world where everything is "supersized". Portions are much larger than they were 20-30 years ago. This is attributed to the obesity epidemic the US is facing. You can take simple steps to make certain you will maintain a healthy weight.

What is portion control?

Portion control is the understanding of exact measures or serving sizes per calorie counts of nutrients for different foods and beverages. Portion control assists in maintaining a healthy body weight. You measure out the right serving size needed to meet your nutritional needs. Again, this is where food labels come in handy. I will also provide you will a list of the 5 main food group foods including the quantity, calories, protein, carbohydrates, and fat per serving. On the next couple of pages you will find several different types of foods in each of the food groups.

Complex Carbohydrate List (Starchy)

- <u>Black Beans</u>: ½ cup (4.6 oz.) 100 calories, 20g carbs, 7g protein, .5g fat
- <u>Whole wheat bread</u>: 1 slice (1 oz.) 90 calories, 20g carbs, 5g protein, 1.5g fat
- <u>Corn</u>: ½ cup (4.6 oz.) 90 calories, 18g carbs, 2g protein, 1g fat
- <u>Oatmeal-steel cut</u>: ¼ cup (1.4 oz.) 150 calories, 27g carbs, 5g protein, 2.5 g fat
- <u>Whole wheat pasta</u>: 1 oz. 105 calories, 20g carbs, 4.5g
  protein, 1g fat
- <u>Peas</u>: ½ cup (2.8 oz.) 60 calories, 11g carbs,4g protein, 0g fat
- <u>Whole wheat Pita bread</u>: 1 large (2.1 oz.) 145 calories, 27g carbs, 6g protein, 1.5g fat
- <u>White potato</u>: 1 large (8 oz.) 210 calories, 49g carbs, 4.4g protein, .2g fat
- <u>Long-grain brown rice</u>: 1 cup (6.9 oz.) 216 calories, 45g carbs, 5g protein, 1.8g fat
- <u>Sweet potato</u>: 1 medium (6 oz.) 136 calories, 31.6g carbs, 2.1g protein, .4g fat
- <u>Quinoa</u>: 1.4 cup (6 oz.) 156 calories, 27.3g carbs, 6g protein, .2g fat
- <u>Yam</u>: 5 oz. 167 calories, 39.5g carbs, 2.2g protein, .2g fat

Complex Carbohydrate-Vegetables (Fibrous)

- <u>Asparagus</u>: 10 7"spears (6.6 oz.) 40 calories, 8g carbs, 4g protein, 0g fat
- <u>Broccoli</u>: 1 cup (3.2 oz.) 30 calories, 4g carbs, 2g protein, 0g fat
- <u>Cabbage</u>: 1 cup chopped (3 oz.) 21 calories, 5g carbs, 1g protein, 0g fat
- <u>Carrots</u>: 1 large (2.8 oz.) 31 calories, 7.3g carbs, .7g protein, .1g fat
- <u>Cauliflower</u>: 1 cup (3.5 oz.) 25 calories, 5g carbs, 2g protein, 0g fat
- <u>Cucumber</u>: 1 small (6 oz.) 20 calories, 4g carbs, 2g protein, 0g fat
- <u>Green beans</u>: 1 cup (4oz) 33 calories, 8g carbs, 2.6g protein, 0g fat
- <u>Romaine lettuce</u>: 3 cups (6oz) 30 calories, 6g carbs, 2g protein, 0g fat
- <u>Onion</u>: ½ cup (2.6 oz.) 30 calories, 6.9g carbs, .9g protein, .1g fat
- <u>Salsa</u>: 4 tablespoons 20 calories, 5g carbs, 0g protein, 0g fat
- <u>Spinach</u>: 3 cups (3 oz.) 20 calories, 3g carbs, 2g protein, 0g fat
- <u>Tomato</u>: 1 medium 25 calories, 6g carbs, 1g protein, 0g fat

Fruit

- <u>Apple</u>: 1 medium (5.4 oz.) 80 calories, 21g carbs, 0g protein, 0g fat
- <u>Banana</u>: 1 medium (4.4 oz.) 110 calories, 29g carbs, 1.0g protein, 0g fat
- <u>Blueberries</u>: 1 cup (5.1 oz.) 82 calories, 20.4g carbs, 1.0g protein, 0g fat
- <u>Cantaloupe</u>: 1 cup diced (5.2 oz.) 53 calories, 13g carbs, 1.3g protein, .3g fat
- <u>Cherries</u>: 1 cup (5.5 oz.) 97 calories, 25g carbs, 1.6g protein, .3g fat
- <u>Grapefruit</u>: 1.2 large (4.7 oz.) 53 calories, 13.4g carbs, 1.1g protein, .2g fat
- <u>Grapes (seedless)</u>: 20 (3.4 oz.) 72 calories, 17.8g carbs, .6g protein, .2g fat
- <u>Mango</u>: 1 cup (5.5 oz.) 99 calories, 25g carbs, 1.4g protein, .6g fat
- <u>Orange</u>: 1 medium (5 oz.) 65 calories, 16.3g carbs, 1.0g protein, .3g fat
- <u>Pear</u>: 1 medium (5.9 oz.) 100 calories, 26g carbs, 1.0g protein, 1 g fat
- <u>Pineapple</u>: 1 cup (5.8 oz.) 82 calories, 22g carbs, 1g protein, 0g fat
- <u>Strawberries</u>: 1 cup (5.4 oz.) 46 calories, 10.6g carbs, 1.0g protein, 0g fat
- <u>Watermelon</u>: 1 cup diced (5.5 oz.) 46 calories, 11g carbs, .9g protein, .2g fat

Lean Proteins

- Ground Beef 90% lean: (4 oz.) 199 calories, 0g carbs, 22.6g protein, 11.3g fat
- Beef top sirloin, lean: (4 oz.) 144 calories, 0g carbs, 34.4g protein, 9.1g fat
- Beef, top round: (4 oz.) 146 calories, 0g carbs, 26.1g protein, 3.8g fat
- Chicken breast, skinless: (4 oz.) 120 calories, 0g carbs, 26g protein, 1.0g fat
- Egg-whole: (1 large) 70 calories, .4g carbs, 6.3g protein, 4.0g fat
- Egg-whites: (1 large) 17 calories, .2g carbs, 3.6g protein, 0g fat
- Fish, salmon: (4 oz.) 206 calories, 0g carbs, 28.8g protein, 9.2g fat
- Fish, tilapia: (4 oz.) 110 calories, 0g carbs, 23g protein, 2.0g fat
- Lobster: (4 oz.) 102 calories, .6g carbs, 21.3g protein, 1.0g fat
- Protein powder Whey: (1 scoop) 120 calories, 2g carbs, 24g protein, 1.0g fat
- Shrimp: (4 oz.) 120 calories, 1g carbs, 23g protein, 2.0g fat
- Turkey breast, skinless: (4oz) 178 calories, 0g carbs, 33.9g protein, 3.7g fat

Dairy

- Cheese, American: 1 slice (1 oz.) 30 calories, 4g carbs, 5g protein, 0g fat
- Cheese, feta low-fat: ½ cup (2 oz.) 120 calories, 0g carbs, 12g protein, 8g fat
- Cheese, Swiss light: 1 slice (1 oz.) 35 calories, 1g carbs, 2g protein, 2g fat
- Cottage cheese, 1% low-fat: ½ cup (4 oz.) 100 calories, 5g carbs, 17.5g protein, 1.3g fat
- Cream cheese, reduced fat: 1/8 package (1 oz.) 70 calories, 1g carbs, 2g protein, 6g fat
- Milk, skim: 1 cup (8 fl oz.) 90 calories, 12g carbs, 8g protein, 0g fat
- Milk, 1%: 1 cup (8 fl oz.) 100 calories, 11g carbs, 8g protein, 2g fat
- Sour cream, nonfat: 2 tablespoons (1.1 oz.) 25 calories, 4g carbs, 2g protein, 0g fat
- Yogurt, fruit, 1% low-fat: 1 (8 oz.) 250 calories, 50g carbs, 9g protein, 2g fat
- Yogurt, non-fat: 1 (8 oz.) 100 calories, 17g carbs, 8g protein, 0g fat
- Yogurt, Greek plain: 1 (6 oz.) 120 calories, 7g carbs, 18g protein, 0g rat
- Yogurt, Greek, vanilla: 1 (6oz) 120 calories, 13g carbs, 16g protein, 0g fat

Planning your meals

Now that you have the fundamental components of the food groups, you can plan your meals for a day, a couple of days, or for the week to ensure you are getting the necessary nutrients needed for optimal health.

In the next several pages you will find sample food menus for the week. Every day is different, but you can prepare ahead if you are short on time; this is called meal prepping. With meal prepping, you cook your meals typically for the week; it can be just your lunch; or lunch, dinner, and your snacks. If you have adequate Tupperware to store the foods, this is an easy and convenient way to save time if you have a busy work week schedule.

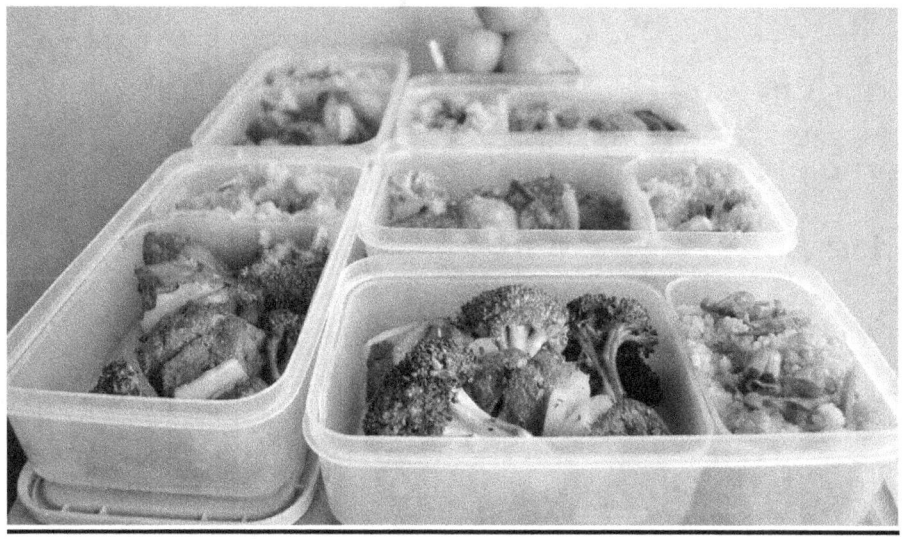

(Meal Prep for 5 days- Lunch)

Sample Menu #1

Breakfast:

2-3 scrambled eggs

1 small orange

2 pieces of whole grain toast

1 cup of skim milk

Mid-Morning Snack: ¼ cup of almonds

Lunch:

Chicken Salad (made by you) with Balsamic Vinaigrette

1 Pear

1 String Cheese

Afternoon Snack: Apple slices with peanut butter

Dinner:

4-6 oz. Grilled chicken breast

1-1 ½ cups brown rice

Steamed broccoli

1 whole wheat dinner roll

Sample Menu #2

Breakfast:

1-1 ½ cups rolled oats (or steel cut)

¼ cup of Blueberries

1 cup Vanilla almond milk

Mid-Morning Snack: 1 Apple and ½ cup of low fat cottage cheese

Lunch:

Peanut Butter and Jelly on whole grain bread

1 cup carrots w/light dip

1 slice of Swiss cheese

Afternoon Snack: ¼ cup of peanuts

Dinner:

4-6 oz. Salmon

Side salad

1 sweet potato

½ cup wild rice

1 cup skim milk

Sample Menu #3

Breakfast:

1-1 ½ cups Greek Yogurt

¼ cup walnuts

1 pear

1 cup Vanilla almond milk

Mid-Morning Snack: whole grain muffin w/jam

Lunch:

Medium Chicken bowl (grilled chicken, brown rice, and broccoli)

2 tbsp. Peanut sauce

1 orange

Afternoon snack: 3-4 cups of popcorn

Dinner:

4-6 oz. Top Sirloin, grilled

1 cup green beans

1 cup Rosemary Red potatoes (diced)

8 oz. Skim Milk

Sample Menu #4

Breakfast:

3 medium pancakes

Sugar-free syrup

2 strips of bacon

1 cup coffee (with Splenda and almond milk)

Mid-Morning snack: 1 cup broccoli with 2 tbsp. light ranch

Lunch:

Turkey Sandwich (whole grain bread, 1 tomato, lettuce, Dijon mustard, 1 slice of cheese)

½ cup unsweetened applesauce

1 string cheese

Afternoon snack: 1 cup strawberries and ½ cup low-fat yogurt

Dinner:

2 cups Chili (93% lean ground beef, red kidney beans, and diced tomatoes)

1 cup brown rice

1 cup French style green beans (no salt added)

Sample Menu #5

Breakfast:

1 whole wheat English muffin

3 strips of turkey bacon

3 egg whites (or 9 tbsp liquid egg whites)

2 cantaloupe slices

Mid-Morning snack: 1 cup sugar snap peas

Lunch:

Taco Salad-with 93% lean ground beef, tomatoes, lettuce, low-fat cheese, 1 Tbsp. light sour cream, ¾ cup baked tortilla chips crushed up.

Afternoon snack: 4 tbsp. Hummus and ½ cucumber

Dinner:

6 oz. grilled Halibut

5-10 spears of Asparagus

1 cup Mashed potatoes

1 whole wheat roll

1 cup Skim milk

Sample Menu #6

Breakfast:

2 whole grain waffles

4 Tbsp. sugar free syrup

1 cup strawberries

1 cup almond milk

Mid-Morning snack: 2 celery sticks with 2 Tbsp. peanut butter

Lunch:

1 Veggie Black Bean burger (no bun with lettuce as your bun)

1 slice tomato

1 Tbsp. ketchup or Dijon mustard

1 Protein shake (2 or less sugars)

Afternoon snack: 1 medium banana

Dinner:

4 oz. baked chicken

1 cup whole wheat pasta

½ cup marinara sauce

1 cup Skim milk

Sample Menu #7

Breakfast:

1 whole grain bagel

2 Tbsp. light cream cheese

1 Grapefruit

Mid-Morning snack: 8 oz. light yogurt

Lunch:

1 cup bean soup

Side salad w/ 2 tbsp. light dressing

1 cup diced pineapple

Mid afternoon snack: 15 baby carrots w/ light dip

Dinner:

4-6 oz. grilled turkey breast

½ cup Quinoa

1 cup Brussel sprouts

1 cup mixed fruit

1 cup skim milk

A Healthy Menu for your Life

When you make small changes toward healthy eating it pays off in many ways. You can lower your risk for certain diseases such as coronary heart disease, diabetes, and obesity; to name a few. Healthy eating is a balancing act. You need a balance of foods from different food groups to ensure you will get all the nutrients your body needs. You need to balance the calories you consume and the amount you exert during exercise to prevent weight gain. Sometimes old habits are hard to break. Take it one day at time. If you find it difficult to give up the foods you love, you can limit the amount you consume by eating less than you normally would. Consume just one serving size of your favorite food.

As you learn to adapt to these new eating skills, you will become better prepared to prevent slips in overindulging and get back on track if they happen.

Chapter 10

Staying Motivated

Whether you have made drastic changes or small improvements to your exercise and eating habits, now is the time to celebrate your successes. You can now look ahead for ways to turn that success into lifelong habits.

In this chapter, you will learn how to overcome barriers to eating and exercise to avoid a relapse. Staying on track can be difficult, but when you feel better, look better, have more energy, and those around you notice all of these wonderful changes you will wonder why you didn't start long ago!

Changing habits aren't easy

Changing our habits can prove to be a difficult task; whether it is improving your eating habits, getting more exercise, losing weight, or even quitting smoking, these changes occur in steps. Think back to time when you thought about changing a habit. What made you want to change? Did you follow through with the change? How long did it take to change that habit? Did you stick to it? If the answer is no, let's find healthy ways to ensure you stick with changing those habits. It took you years to develop those habits, so give yourself time to make the adjustments necessary to develop a healthier way of eating and exercising.

Focus on the Positive

Our minds play a powerful role in how we look at things. When you focus on the positive, you have positive results; even if it is minimal. If you focus on the negative, you will have negative results.

To keep you motivated, below is list of several small successes you can focus on:

- Tried something new
- Achieved a short term goal
- Exercised for 30 minutes, 5 times this week
- Made healthy meals in advance to save time
- Noticed improvements in my mood
- Kept a food log much of the time
- Made improvements in food portions
- Drank water instead of soda
- Ate one of my favorite meals and didn't feel guilty
- I feel better when I exercise
- I feel better when I make healthy eating choices
- Became a smarter grocery shopper
- Noticed improvements in self-esteem or confidence
- Made healthier choices when eating out
- Improvement in overall health (lower blood pressure, lowered cholesterol, or reduced medications)
- Improved my ability to control my eating triggers
- I no longer get short of breath during exercise
- NSV (non-scale victories) improvement in strength, more energy, clothes fit better, you are eating more vegetables and drinking more water.

- Helped others to make changes in eating habits

It's a Learning Process

We all have to start somewhere. Think of it like school; you started in Kindergarten and worked your way up to graduating High School. It took many years for you to learn everything you know now. It is the same when you begin to learn new habits in diet and exercise. You may hit a snag along the way, and that is normal part of the process. *The key is to never give up.*

Identify Barriers

Another key process in staying motivated is identifying barriers that may have inhibited your past successes with diet and exercise. A barrier is anything that could get in your way of making successful changes. Now ask yourself, what are some factors that kept you from eating a healthy diet? What were the reasons you didn't get physical activity for at least 30 minutes each day?

That first step is to identify the problem. Choose one of your personal barriers and think through it thoroughly. For example, you have a family gathering that prevents you from eating healthy or you find you consume far more than the amount of calories you should. Try to remember the events of that family gathering. What specific thoughts or actions seemed to get in the way of healthy eating goals? Were you too busy to prepare healthy meals? Did you feel pressured by family to eat that second or even third helping of food? Did your grandmother specifically make your favorite cake just for you and felt obligated to eat more than one piece? The more specific you can describe the problem, the more focused you will be to have a healthy solution.

Develop Solutions

Once you have identified your barriers, it is now up to you to develop solutions to prevent a lapse in your new journey to a healthier you. To better assist you, below is a list of common barriers to diet and exercise and potential solutions:

1. **No Time-** This really is just an excuse. If you really want to do something, you will make the time. If you find that preparing your lunch for the next day in the morning you have to work is time consuming, make your meal the night before, so you can grab and go. If time is factor as to why you don't exercise, spread out your exercise during the day. Wake up 10 minutes early and go for a quick run. During your lunch break, walk around your office building or maybe a mall is nearby you can get your exercise walking the mall.

2. **Healthy Food is Expensive-** It really isn't. If you shop at stores like Sprouts, or your local farmer's market, the produce is usually less expensive than the typical grocery store. If you buy Organic, yes, it is more expensive. If you don't buy Organic, you can easily wash your food before you prepare it. Packaged items are more expensive than those you would find at the grocery store, but if you can buy food in its most natural form, that will give you your best benefit.

3. **Grazing at Family Gatherings**- This is a big one. You have your entire family together and there is all but food around you. You talk and eat. Next thing you know, several hours have gone by and you ate that entire time! You have to really discipline yourself to not eat because others around you are eating. Grab a glass of water instead. Make a small plate instead of grabbing here and there at the different foods.

4. **Lack of Social Support**- Maybe you want to change your habits and start eating healthy and exercise, but you have a spouse or friends who are not as supportive. They may see you as their "drinking buddy", why would you want to get in shape now? You have an unsupportive spouse who may fear that if you lose weight and feel better about yourself, they may see it as a threat that you will leave. Maybe you do not have family close to talk to and they do not have the same views as you. This can really hinder your motivation.

   Today there are so many groups online that have perfect strangers who will root you on! Also, local social groups you can become a part of to help you in your diet and exercise journey.

5. **Stressful Job**- This is where getting exercise comes in handy! Even if you work a 12 hour day, take just 10 minutes a day to get exercise at home. If you have a gym membership, take advantage of it! If you work late into

the afternoon, go to the gym in the morning. This means going to bed earlier than you normally would. Getting exercise is a great stress reliever! If there is no way you will go to the gym in the early morning, refer back to my home workout in Chapter 6.

6. **You don't like "healthy foods"-** You have always been a picky eater or you grew up eating fast food or food in box. Old habits are hard to break, but you can break them! Take is slow and give it time. Maybe you don't like certain foods because you have never tried them before. You don't want to give up your favorite foods completely, but you may need to change how often you eat them. Introduce new dishes once a week or every other week and try new foods. It can take several months to adjust to a new way of eating, but you can do it!

These are just a few examples that might apply to you. Add to the list as you need and don't forget to ask yourself "what and why" when it comes to your barriers and answer "how" you will overcome them.

Reward Yourself

You are putting in 100% effort in your eating habits and change in exercise for the better. There is nothing more motivating than giving yourself a reward for all your hard work! And by reward, I do not necessarily mean food rewards but I won't discredit them either. Non-food rewards can also be motivating to help you continue on with your journey to health and fitness.

Non-Food Rewards

1. Buy new clothes- You've lost 40 pounds and now all of your clothes don't fit! The greatest victory is fitting into a size you did when you were in high school.

2. Get a massage- Adding strength training to your workout can cause sore muscles and a massage will soothe them!

3. Subscribe to fitness or cooking healthy magazine- Everyone could use help in new ideas and maybe you can introduce a family member or friend to a new healthy recipe you've discovered.

4. Get a new hairstyle- New body, new you! You will feel great after you get your hair done at the salon. A great confidence booster.

5. Buy a pedometer- investing in a fitness tracker can motivate you even more! A pedometer tracks the amount of steps you take in a day. Some pedometers even track your sleep patterns if you wear them at night (ex. Fitbit).

6. Take a mini vacation- Head up to the mountains for a weekend hike, or to the beach and relax.

Rewards don't have to be expensive. You could by books from a used book store and clothes from a second hand store (especially if you are planning to drop more sizes). There are also rewards that do not cost a thing. Examples are a candle-lit bubble bath at home alone, laying down for a nap, or just enjoy the peace and quiet.

You can also set up a system where you can earn rewards as you achieve daily and weekly goals. Keep a log in a place where you will see it every day. Give yourself a "gold" star for every task you complete and earn your reward. It can help get you motivated to do even more!

Food Rewards- The good and the bad

Adopting new eating and exercise habits take time and patience, but rewarding yourself with your favorite cake or candy isn't always the best choice. What begins to happen is you complete a goal, (let's say you lost 5 pounds, now you think it is okay to eat that cake) you look to food as your reward for this accomplishment. Then you feel guilty because you didn't just eat one piece cake but four pieces; there goes that 5 pound victory. I am not saying this will happen to you, but it is highly likely. It can be easy to revert back to your old ways.

The good with food rewards is that they don't have to be the unhealthiest item you could possibly eat. You can reward yourself with strawberries and whip cream; just enough sweet to curb your cravings. You can still eat a tasty treat and save on the calories.

The Final Take

Making lasting changes in your diet and fitness will take time, it doesn't happen overnight. You have to be patient and understand that there are no quick fixes. You didn't decide one day that you wanted to gain 50 pounds, it happened over time. The same goes for weight loss. It could take 6 months or longer to lose 40 pounds. Changing your eating habits from mindless eating to conscious eating is a gradual process, and you will get off track now and again. Life happens to all of us. We grow as individuals and we learn new ways of doing things. It is not always easy. The key to a healthy you is finding a balance between diet and exercise. You will find it to be easier to develop lasting healthy habits if you slowly incorporate fitness and eating right rather than going in full force ahead. This will set you up for failure. So remember to start low and go slow.

The accomplishment of a healthy and happy you are the greatest reward anyone could ask for!

Additional Resources

1. www.webmd.com

2. www.cdc.gov

3. www.health.gov

4. www.heart.gov

5. www.nutritiondata.com

6. www.fda.gov

7. www.choosemyplate.gov

8. www.myfitnesspal.com

9. www.usda.gov

About the Author

Renee Chatham, C.P.T.

Born in Northwest Indiana, Renee moved to Colorado with her only daughter in 1999; this is where she developed a passion for fitness and health. Renee dedicated nearly every day to exercise and eating right. She also lost her mother to breast cancer at an early age and wanted to be as healthy as she could for her own daughter.

After 14 years of fitness and exercise on her own, Renee decided she wanted to help others achieve fitness success and became a certified personal trainer. Renee dedicated every minute to learning as much as she possibly could; and with two years in, she collected twelve additional specialties in fitness. A few of those include; weight loss, women's fitness, senior fitness, sports injury, orthopedic exercise, and fitness nutrition coach, just to name a few.

Renee has been helping others win their battle with healthy eating and exercise since 2013. Renee's first publication was for a local magazine; an article about outdoor fitness for *Southlands Life* magazine in 2014. She hopes to continue to inspire and motivate as many people as she possibly can through fitness in the years to come.

For more information visit: **www.optfitness-1.com**

Index

www.ingramcontent.com/pod-product-compliance
Lightning Source LLC
Chambersburg PA
CBHW081107290526
45795CB00006B/2035